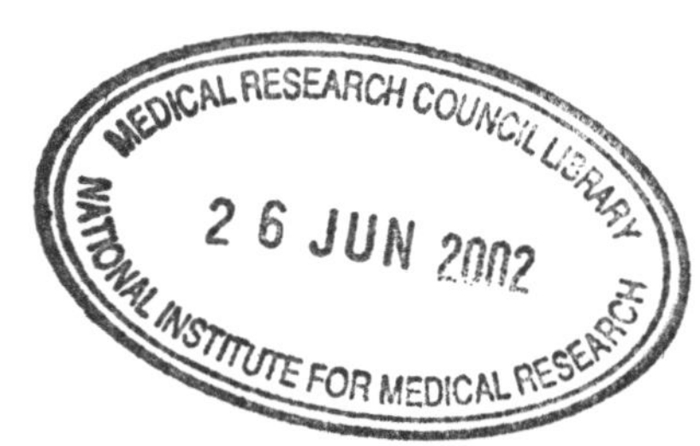

Keio University International Symposia
for Life Sciences and Medicine 9

Springer

Tokyo
Berlin
Heidelberg
New York
Barcelona
Hong Kong
London
Milan
Paris

M. Kitajima, M. Shimazu,
G. Wakabayashi, K. Hoshino,
M. Tanabe, S. Kawachi (Eds.)

Current Issues in Liver and Small Bowel Transplantation

With 46 Figures

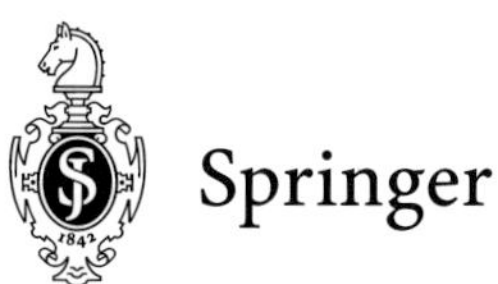

Springer

Masaki Kitajima, M.D.
Motohide Shimazu, M.D.
Go Wakabayashi, M.D.
Ken Hoshino, M.D.
Minoru Tanabe, M.D.
Shigeyuki Kawachi, M.D.

Department of Surgery
School of Medicine, Keio University
35 Shinanomachi, Shinjuku-ku
Tokyo 160-8582, Japan

ISBN 4-431-70332-2 Springer-Verlag Tokyo Berlin Heidelberg New York

Library of Congress Cataloging-in-Publication Data Applied for

Printed on acid-free paper

Typesetting: SNP Best-set Typesetter Ltd., Hong Kong
Printing and binding: Hicom, Japan
SPIN: 10832970

Foreword

This volume of the Keio University International Symposia for Life Sciences and Medicine contains the proceedings of the ninth symposium held under the sponsorship of the Keio University Medical Science Fund. As explained in the Opening Remarks by the President of Keio University, the fund was established by the generous donation of Dr. Mitsunada Sakaguchi. The Keio University International Symposia for Life Sciences and Medicine constitute one of the core activities sponsored by the fund, the objective of which is to contribute to the international community by developing human resources, promoting scientific knowledge, and encouraging mutual exchange. Each year, the Committee of the International Symposia for Life Sciences and Medicine selects the most significant symposium topic from applications received from the Keio medical community. The publication of the proceedings is intended to publicize and disseminate the information arising from the lively discussions of the most exciting and current issues presented during the symposium. On behalf of the Committee, I am most grateful to Dr. Mitsunada Sakaguchi, who made the symposia series possible. We are also grateful to the prominent speakers for their contribution to this volume. In addition, we would like to acknowledge the efficient organizational work performed by the members of the program committee and the staff of the fund.

Naoki Aikawa, M.D., D.M.Sc., F.A.C.S.
Chairman
Committee of the International Symposia
for Life Sciences and Medicine

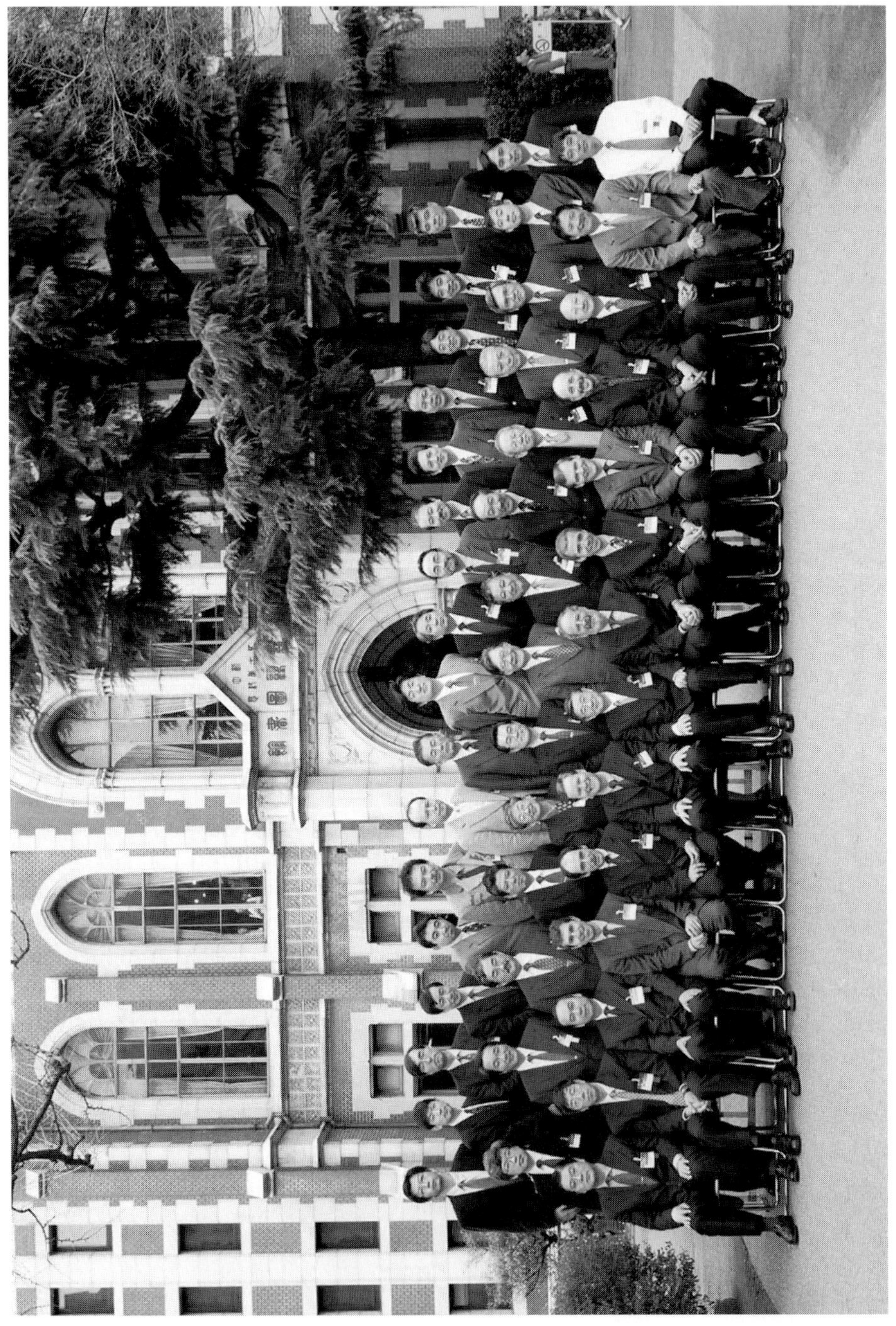

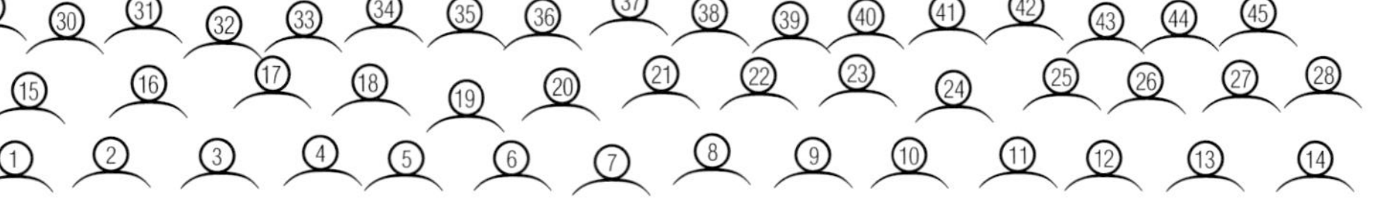

The 9th Keio University International Symposium for Life Sciences and Medicine

Speakers, chairpersons, and discussants at the symposium are identified in the photograph by numbers on the diagram.

1. Seiichi Suzuki 2. Sung Gyu Lee 3. Chao-Long Chen 4. René Adam 5. Olivier Goulet 6. Peter Neuhaus 7. Masaki Kitajima
8. Gary A. Levy 9. Xavier Rogiers 10. Björn Nashan 11. Alan N. Langnas 12. Sheung-Tat Fan 13. John J. Fung 14. Seigo Nishida
16. Namiki Izumi 17. Kazunori Aso 18. Susumu Satomi 19. Sachiyo Suita 20. Morito Monden 21. Hiromasa Ishii 22. Kenji Fujiwara
23. Takafumi Ichida 24. Kunio Okuda 25. Shozo Baba 26. Toshifumi Hibi 27. Yukihiro Inomata 28. Minoru Tanabe
34. Hidetoshi Matsunami 35. Tatsuto Ashizawa 39. Takashi Hashimoto 40. Motohide Shimazu 41. Atsushi Sugioka
42. Go Wakabayashi 43. Ken Hoshino 44. Hidetsugu Saito 45. Hiromichi Ikawa

Preface

In Japan, cadaveric donor liver transplantation is not common even though cadaveric organ transplantation was legally established in 1998. In contrast, the number of living donor liver transplantations is increasing, with more than 1700 cases at 43 Japanese institutes by November 2001. Indications for living donor liver transplantation are widening in Japan and have become similar to those for cadaveric donor liver transplantation in the United States and Europe. At the same time, split liver transplantation from cadaveric donors shares some technical aspects with living donor liver transplantation. Remarkable progress has been reported recently, and thus it was an auspicious time to hold a symposium on "Current issues in liver/small bowel transplantation" in Japan.

We were honored to hold a very fruitful symposium sponsored by the Keio University Medical Science Fund and to bring together top-rank transplant surgeons from Japan and other countries. It was a productive and rewarding time for all participants. We were able to share our experience through excellent presentations followed by active discussions and insightful comments. At the symposium, we focused on current issues in liver transplantation such as widening indications for viral hepatitis and malignant tumors. We also discussed technical aspects and physiological problems in split/living donor liver transplant, novel strategies in immunosuppression, and the current status and future prospects in small bowel transplantation. This book contains the papers from all the distinguished guest speakers, focusing on the topics discussed at the symposium.

It has been a year since the symposium ended; however, the topics we discussed are still very important and the papers in this book remain informative to all who are working in this field. The editors are grateful to the distinguished guest speakers for submitting their important papers for publication in this volume. We would like to take this opportunity to express our deep gratitude to Dr. Mitsunada Sakaguchi, an alumnus of the School of Medicine, Keio University, for his generous donation that made possible the creation of the Keio University Medical Science Fund.

February 2002
Masaki Kitajima
Motohide Shimazu
Go Wakabayashi

Contents

Part 1 Technical Aspects and Physiological Problems in Split/Living Donor Liver Transplantation

List of Contributors

Opening Remarks

Prof. Yasuhiko Torii
President, Keio University
Chairman, Keio University Medical Science Fund

Ladies and Gentlemen:

On behalf of the whole of Keio University, I have very great pleasure in welcoming you all to the 9th Keio University International Symposium for Life Sciences and Medicine. I am particularly grateful to the distinguished scientists who have traveled such long distances to participate in this meeting.

The topic of our symposium this year is Current Issues in Liver/Small Bowel Transplantation. Although remarkable progress and breakthroughs are reported almost every day in the field of organ transplantation, it is also true that there are still many who suffer from end-stage liver and small bowel disease. The present time therefore seems an opportune moment to hold a related symposium at Keio University, and all speakers kindly accepted our invitation to contribute to a symposium on Liver/Small Bowel Transplantation. I feel certain that this unique meeting will prove both exciting and successful.

Keio University, the oldest university among the 604 universities in Japan, was founded in 1858 by Yukichi Fukuzawa. He was a pioneer of modern civilization in Japan. Fukuzawa was a member of the very first mission of the Tokugawa Shogunate government to the United States in 1860 and to European countries in 1862. Before that time, the Shogun had closed Japan's doors to the outside world in a period of self-isolation lasting almost 300 years, until the American Admiral Perry knocked on our door. Fukuzawa realized during his visits to the United States and Europe as a member of the official Japanese mission that education was crucially important to the future of Japan. How highly his achievements were valued by the Japanese Government is reflected in the fact that his portrait is printed on the Japanese 10,000 yen bank note. Thus, Keio has its origins in international exchanges: indeed, international exchanges such as this symposium have been one of the most important academic and social missions of Keio University since its foundation.

In the fall of 1994, Dr. Mitsunada Sakaguchi, an alumnus of the 1940 class of our medical school, donated five billion yen to the university. He expressed the wish that his fund should be used to encourage research in life sciences and medicine at Keio University and to promote worldwide advancements in science. I fully agreed with his proposal, and thus launched the Keio University Medical Science Fund in April 1995. The International Symposium for Life Sciences and Medicine has been organized as one of several projects supported by the fund. In 1999, Dr. Sakaguchi made an additional donation of two billion yen.

We are now witnessing the dawn of the 21st century and the third millennium. We realize that society faces many problems that will be carried over into the new century. Many new and unknown difficulties also await us. I believe that exploring new horizons in life sciences is one of the most vital tasks facing us at the dawn of the 21st century. It is equally important to ensure that the knowledge gained through such pursuits will be used in a way that brings genuine happiness to humankind.

It is thus more than a pleasure, indeed it is an honor, for me to be able to meet the distinguished medical researchers and clinicians from world-renowned institutions gathered here, and to share in a frank and valuable exchange of views. I am also grateful for the efforts made by the organizing committee, chaired by Dr. Masaki Kitajima, who has devoted himself to ensuring that this symposium is an auspicious and enjoyable event. I do hope that the meeting will prove a truly fruitful and productive one for you all.

Let me close by wishing everyone gathered here further success in their research and clinical work. Thank you very much.

Part 1
Technical Aspects and Physiological Problems in Split/Living Donor Liver Transplantation

Living-Donor Liver Transplantation: Experience at Shinshu University

Seiji Kawasaki

Summary. We have performed 143 living-donor liver transplantations (LDLTs) on 143 patients (83 pediatric and 60 adult patients). The type of donor hepatectomy in pediatric cases was left lateral segmentectomy in 50 cases, extended lateral segmentectomy in 20 cases, and left lobectomy in 13 cases, while in adult cases we carried out left lobectomy in 58 cases (combined left-side caudate lobectomy in 8 cases), right posterior segmentectomy in 1 case, and right lobectomy in 1 case (a patient with familial amyloidosis in a domino transplantation). In 2 of the 58 cases using a left lobar graft, temporary auxiliary transplantation was performed since the donor's left lobe was disproportionately small. No banked blood was transfused in any living-related donor. The postoperative course of all living-related donors was uneventful, without any major complications or reoperation. The survival rates after 1 and 5 years in these 143 patients were 87% and 84%, respectively. The results were comparable between pediatric and adult patients, although the implanted graft was significantly small-for-size in adult cases.

Key words. Living-related transplantation, Auxiliary transplantation, Domino transplantation, Small-for-size graft

In Japan, 40000 people die of chronic liver disease annually. It is estimated that liver transplantation is indicated for 3000 of these 40000. However, cadaveric liver transplantation faced with legal difficulties until 1997, when a law was passed setting the legal basis by which organ transplantations from brain-dead donors can be performed. Even though the law took effect, only a few cadaveric liver transplantations have been carried out to date [1]. The only

First Department of Surgery, Shinshu University School of Medicine, 3-1-1 Asahi, Matsumoto 390-8621, Japan alternative at present is living-donor liver transplantation (LDLT). Since 1989, LDLT has been performed in pediatric patients in several institutions in Japan with good results, although it was initially considered that this surgical procedure could not be applied to adult patients.

We reported the first successful case of an adult-to-adult LDLT, using a whole left lobar graft including the middle hepatic vein, in 1994 [2]. This led us to believe that LDLT would become an indispensable treatment modality for adult patients with end-stage liver disease because the number of adult patients accounts for more than 85% of all patients who need liver transplantation. Adult patients also suffer greatly from donor scarcity in Western countries, where cadaveric liver transplantation programs have already been established. Since then we have performed LDLTs for both pediatric and adult patients using left-side liver grafts in most cases [3, 4]. This chapter describes our experience with LDLT.

Patients and Methods

Recipients

Between June 1990 and March 2001, we performed 143 LDLTs on 143 patients: 83 pediatric cases and 60 adults. In the pediatric patients, the underlying diseases were biliary atresia in 59, fulminant hepatic failure in 13, Alagille's syndrome in 5, neonatal hepatitis in 2, and primary sclerosing cholangitis, late-onset hepatic failure, Wilson's disease, and Byler's disease in 1 each. The underlying diseases in adult cases were familial amyloid polyneuropathy in 15, primary biliary cirrhosis in 14, liver cirrhosis secondary to hepatitis B or C in 9, citrullinemia in 7, fulminant hepatic failure in 6, primary sclerosing cholangitis in 4, biliary atresia in 2, and glycogen storage disease, Caroli's disease, and autoimmune hepatitis in 1 each. The ages of the pediatric patients ranged from 4 months to 15 years, and the ages of the adult patients ranged from 18 to 69 years.

Donors

The 83 donors in the pediatric cases ranged in age from 20 to 54 years, while the ages of the 60 donors in the adult-to-adult cases ranged from 20 to 61 years. The relationship to the recipient in each case is shown in Table 1. Two domino LDLTs were performed, where the two donors were patients with familial amyloid polyneuropathy (FAP) and were unrelated to the recipients. Each living-related donor was healthy with no hematological or biochemical abnormalities. The donors' packed blood cells (400–800 ml) and fresh-frozen plasma (800–2400 ml) were stored before surgery for possible perioperative

TABLE 1. Donors in 143 cases of living-donor liver transplantation

Relationship	Donors in pediatric cases	Donors in adult cases
Mother	47	7
Father	34	9
Husband	–	10
Son	–	15
Daughter	–	4
Brother	1	5
Sister	–	7
Grandmother	1	–
Nephew	–	1
Unrelated (domino)	–	2
Total	83	60

autotransfusion except for the donors who underwent partial hepatectomy for the recipients with fulminant hepatic failure.

Preoperative Estimation of Graft Volume

The predicted volume of the graft was estimated preoperatively with computed tomography (CT) scan images, as described previously [5]. The standard liver volume in the recipients was calculated from body surface area [6]. The ratio between the graft volume and the standard liver volume (GV/SV ratio) was then calculated. We have accepted donor–recipient combinations giving predicted GV/SV ratios of equal to or more than 30%.

Surgery

In pediatric cases, we performed three types of liver resection for the donor hepatectomy [7]: left lateral segmentectomy in 50 donors, extended lateral segmentectomy in 20 donors, and left lobectomy including the middle hepatic vein in 13 donors. The types of donor hepatectomy in adult-to-adult cases were left lobectomy including the middle hepatic vein in 50 donors, and, left lobectomy including the middle hepatic vein and left-side caudate lobe in 8 donors in whom the predicted GV/SV ratio did not reach 30% without that lobe [8]. In the remaining 2 adult cases, the right posterior segment was obtained from the living-related donor in 1 case in which the left lobar graft could not be used since the donor had a right-sided round ligament. In the other case, the right lobe was used in a graft obtained from a patient with FAP (domino transplantation). The recipient hepatectomy was performed by preserving the inferior vena cava in a way similar to piggyback liver transplantation. In the 2 patients with FAP, a temporary auxiliary partial orthotopic transplantation (APOLT) was performed, with the recipient's right lobe being preserved because the donor's left lobe was disproportionately small. At the time of APOLT in these 2 patients, the right portal vein was ligated and resected to induce atrophy of the right lobe of the native liver and compensatory hypertrophy of the grafted left lobe. Implantation procedures were carried out as described previously [3]. Hepatic arterial reconstruction was carried out under microscopic observation. In patients whose native liver was noncirrhotic, a temporary end-to-side shunt between the right portal vein and the inferior vena cava was made instead of the conventional venovenous bypass during the anhepatic phase to avoid congestion of the portal venous system [9].

Results

The intraoperative blood loss during donor hepatectomy was insignificant in all cases, and no banked blood or blood derivatives were transfused in any living-related donor. The postoperative course in all the 141 living-related donors was basically uneventful, and no donor needed reoperation.

The actual graft volume and GV/SV ratio ranged from 230 ml to 625 ml and from 22% to 65%, respectively, at the time of transplantation in the 60 adult cases (Figs. 1 and 2), while in the 83 pediatric cases the graft volume and GV/SV ratio were in the ranges 165–530 ml and 39%–192%, respectively.

The actual graft volumes in 8 cases in which the left lobe plus left-side caudate lobe were implanted are shown in Table 2. The volumes were 45–105 ml larger than that of segments 2–4 (left lobe without caudate lobe) estimated preoperatively. In the 2 patients who underwent temporary APOLT, the right lobe of the native liver was removed on postoperative days 50 and 63

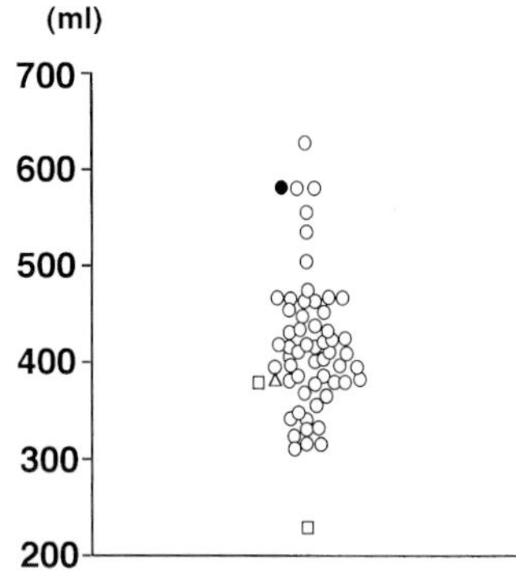

FIG. 1. Graft volume in 60 adult-to-adult cases at the time of transplantation (range 230–625 ml). *Open circles*, left lobar graft; *solid circle*, right lobar graft; *squares*, left lobar graft in temporary auxiliary transplantation; *triangle*, right posterior segmental graft

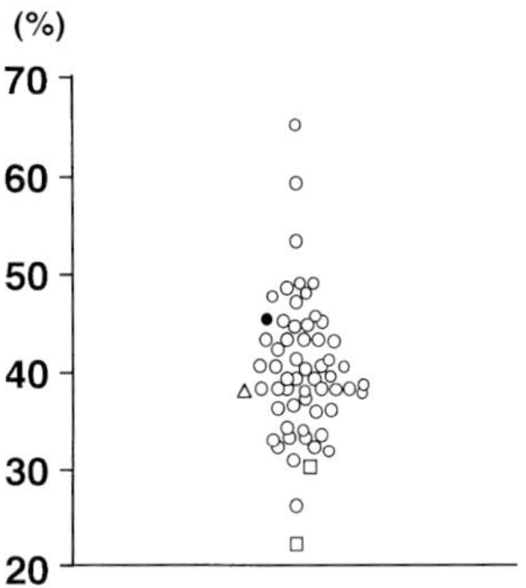

FIG. 2. Ratio of graft volume to standard liver volume (GV/SV) in 60 adult-to-adult cases at the time of transplantation (range 22%–65%). *Open circles*, left lobar graft; *solid circle*, right lobar graft; *squares*, left lobar graft in temporary auxiliary transplantation; *triangle*, right posterior segmental graft

TABLE 2. Eight cases in which the left lobe plus left-side caudate lobe were transplanted

Case	Predicted volume of segments 2–4 (ml)	Actual volume of segments 2–4 plus left-side caudate lobe (ml)
1	315	420
2	315	415
3	347	420
4	286	359
5	300	375
6	260	343
7	311	398
8	355	400

after its atrophy and compensatory hypertrophy of the grafted left lobe had been identified on CT scan images.

The patient whose grafted liver was the smallest (GV/SV ratio 26%), except for the temporary APOLT cases, showed good recovery without significant liver dysfunction (peak level of serum total bilirubin 4.0 mg/dl).

The survival rates of all 143 patients were 87% at 1 year and 84% at 5 years (Fig. 3). No significant difference in the survival rate was observed between pediatric and adult patients (Fig. 4).

Discussion

In January 1999, a national survey of the results of LDLT was conducted by collecting data from institutions all over Japan. This showed that 614 and 180 LDLTs had been performed in pediatric and adult patients, respectively. The survival rate of adult patients was 73.9% at the time of the survey, which is slightly worse than that of pediatric patients at 82.6%. It should be noted that

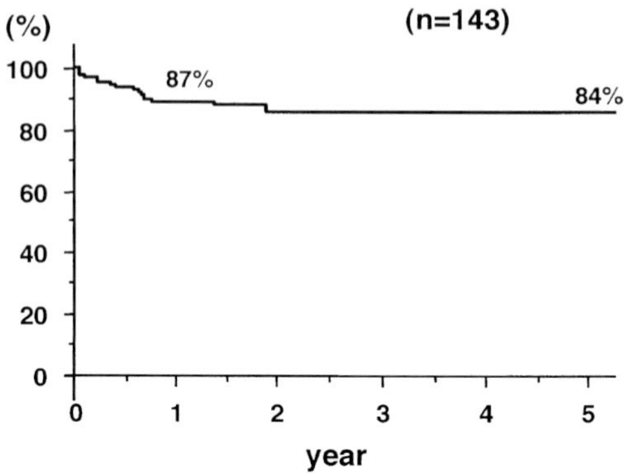

Fig. 3. Graft survival of all 143 patients after living-donor liver transplantion (Kaplan-Meier method)

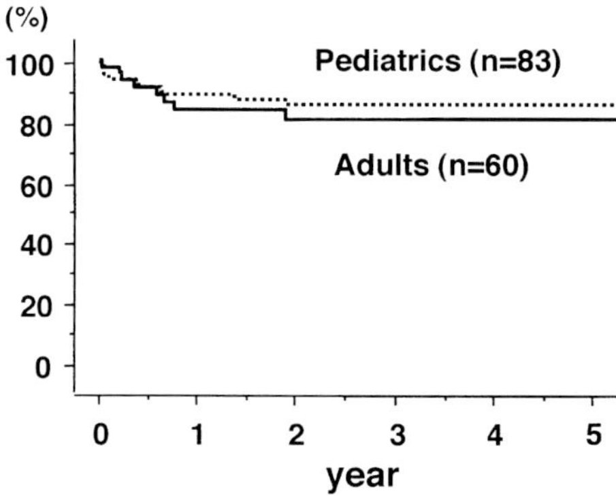

Fig. 4. Graft survival of 83 pediatric and 60 adult patients after living-donor liver transplantion (Kaplan-Meier method)

there is no simple method of comparing the outcome of adult patient, with that of pediatric patients, because the median follow-up in adult patients (probably less than 1 year) was much shorter than that in pediatric recipients. The major reason for this unfavorable outcome for adult patients in Japan is probably related to small-for-size grafting. The volume of the left lobe corresponds to about one-third of the whole liver volume, and in the majority of cases of adult-to-adult LDLT a left lobar graft had been performed before this survey. In 1997, a Hong Kong group reported good results with adult-to-adult LDLT using an extended right lobar graft in seven patients with fulminant hepatic failure [10]. Recently, some institutions in Japan, including Kyoto University, Hokkaido University, and the University of Tokyo, and some institutions in the USA, Europe, and Asia have started an adult-to-adult LDLT program using a right lobar graft [11–13]. At present, the right lobe is being used as a graft in the majority of cases of adult-to-adult LDLT worldwide. In contrast to this worldwide trend, we have not used a right lobe as a graft from a living-related donor because the donor risk would be higher if a right lobectomy were performed rather than a left lobectomy, and we are not positive that this is justified in donor hepatectomy. Therefore, in adult or adolescent cases, the graft to be implanted in our series is inevitably small-for-size. Our criteria for proceeding with LDLT in the present series was that the predicted GV/SV ratio was equal to or more than 30%, although the actual GV/SV ratios included values less than 30% (see Fig. 2). If the recipient receives a left lobar graft obtained from a donor with the same body size, it is likely that the GV/SV ratio at the time of transplantation would be about one-third, i.e., 33%, suggesting that LDLT can be performed for donor–recipient combinations with the same body size on the basis of our criteria. However, the shape of the liver is variable, and the left lobar volume may correspond to less than 30% of the whole liver volume. We have recently started LDLT using a left lobar graft combined with the left-side caudate lobe when the estimated left lobar volume corresponds to less than 30% of recipient's standard liver volume [8]. This new procedure has enabled us to accept the majority of donor–recipients combinations for LDLT from the viewpoint of graft size.

Although the recipient risk would naturally be higher if the left lobe were used as a graft in adult-to-adult LDLT rather than the right lobe, we have set our criteria in terms of graft size for adult-to-adult LDLT and obtained an outcome using a left lobar graft which is comparable with that in pediatric cases.

References

1. Kawasaki S, Hashikura Y, Ikegami T, et al. (1999) First case of cadaveric liver transplantation in Japan. J Hepatobiliary Pancreat Surg 6:387–390
2. Hashikura Y, Makuuchi M, Kawasaki S, et al. (1994) Successful living-related partial liver transplantation to an adult patient. Lancet 343:1233–1234
3. Kawasaki S, Makuuchi M, Matsunami H, et al. (1998) Living-related liver transplantation in adults. Ann Surg 227:269–274
4. Hashikura Y, Kawasaki S, Terada M, et al. (2001) Long-term results of living-related donor liver graft transplantation: a single-center analysis of 110 transplants. Transplantation 72:95–99
5. Kawasaki S, Makuuchi M, Matsunami H, et al. (1993) Preoperative measurement of segmental liver volume of donors for living-related liver transplantation. Hepatology 18:1115–1120
6. Urata K, Kawasaki S, Matsunami H, et al. (1995) Calculation of child and adult standard liver volume for liver transplantation. Hepatology 21:1317–1321
7. Makuuchi M, Kawasaki S, Noguchi T, et al. (1993) Donor hepatectomy for living-related partial liver transplantation. Surgery 113:395–402
8. Miyagawa S, Hashikura Y, Miwa S, et al. (1998) Concomitant caudate lobe resection as an option for donor hepatectomy in adult living-related liver transplantation. Transplantation 66:661–663
9. Kawasaki S, Hashikura Y, Matsunami H, et al. (1996) Temporary shunt between right portal vein and vena cava in living-related liver transplantation. J Am Coll Surg 183:74–76

10. Lo CM, Fan ST, Liu CL, et al. (1997) Adult-to-adult living-related liver transplantation using extended right lobe grafts. Ann Surg 226:261–270
11. Wachs ME, Bak TE, Karrer FM, et al. (1998) Adult living-donor liver transplantation using a right hepatic lobe. Transplantation 66:1313–1316
12. Marcos A, Fisher RA, Ham JM, et al. (1999) Right lobe living donor liver transplantation. Transplantation 68:798–803
13. Kiuchi T, Inomata Y, Uemoto S, et al. (2000) Evolution of living donor liver transplantation in adults: a single center experience. Transplant Int 13(Suppl):S134–135

Liver Splitting for Two Adult Patients and Domino Liver Transplantation: The Paul Brousse Experience

R. Adam, D. Azoulay, D. Castaing, Y.M. Bao, E. Savier,
D. Samuel, and H. Bismuth

The reliability of splitting livers for transplantation into two adult recipients remains to be proven. The aim of this paper was to report our experience with such splitting in two adults. Ex situ and in situ splitting were performed in 15 and 2 cases, respectively, generating 34 grafts (30 transplanted in our center, 4 shipped to two partner centers). Cold ischemia time, intraoperative transfusion volume, and hospitalization stay were comparable for recipients of left and right grafts. Within 15 days of transplantation, liver function tests were significantly better for recipients of right grafts than for recipients of left grafts. Primary nonfunction occurred in three cases and was statistically related to the presence of a graft/body weight ratio (GBWR) of <1% ($P <$ 0.001). Eleven technical complications occurred in eight patients (morbidity rate 24%) including biliary stenosis (four cases); biliary leak and portal vein thrombosis (two cases each); hepatic artery stenosis, subphrenic abscess, and hemoperitoneum (one case each). These complications led to graft loss in three cases, with death resulting in two. After a mean follow-up of 34 months, 24 of 34 patients are alive with normal liver function tests. Actuarial 1-year patient and graft survival rates were, respectively, 80% and 74% for the whole series. Actuarial 1-year patient and graft survival rates for right and left grafts were not statistically different (72% vs. 87% and 72% vs. 76% respectively). We concluded that liver splitting is feasible, but technical progress is needed to increase the reliability of the technique. We also examined the possibility of using domino liver transplants for metabolic disorders, specifically familial amyloidotic polyneuropathy (FAP). The shortage of donors means that new methods of liver procurement must be explored. With domino transplantation, an organ explanted during transplantation in one patient is used for transplantation in a second patient. Domino procedures can be performed

Hôpital Paul Brousse, Villejuif, France

with livers from patients given transplants for hepatic metabolic disorders that cause systemic disease without affecting other liver function. Familial amyloidotic polyneuropathy (FAP) type I is an example. We reviewed our experience with a domino liver transplant program for FAP with a view to extending the approach to other metabolic disorders. Livers from 14 patients given transplants for FAP type 1 were used for domino transplants in 16 patients (two FAP livers were split) with unresectable primary or metastatic liver cancer. There was no perioperative mortality. Neuropathy or cardiomyopathy did not increase the morbidity of the domino liver explant/transplant procedures. The morbidity for the domino recipients did not appear to be increased. One intensive care unit (ICU)-bound recipient of a FAP hemiliver died within 60 days of transplantation. Variant TTR (a marker of FAP disease) was detected in the serum in FAP liver recipients, with no immediate clinical consequences. We concluded that the domino approach is feasible and requires careful planning of the surgical procedures for liver explantation, particularly regarding the nature and site of vascular anastomoses. Domino transplantation of metabolically dysfunctional livers creates new categories of potential donors and potential recipients. It also raises new ethical, technical, and societal issues. The domino approach could be used for several genetic or biochemical disorders now treated by liver transplantation. It has the potential to increase the number of organs available for patients with primary or metastatic liver cancer.

Living-Donor Liver Transplantation in Taiwan

Yaw-Sen Chen, Chao-Long Chen, Vanessa H. de Villa,
Chih-Chi Wang, Shih-Ho Wang, Po-Ping Liu, Yu-Fan Cheng,
Tung-Liang Huang, Bruno Jawan, and Hock-Liew Eng

Summary. Living-donor liver transplantation (LDLT) is currently the only effective means to significantly increase the graft supply in societies where cadaveric donation is very limited, as in Taiwan. Since the Kaohsiung Chang Gung Memorial Hospital (CGMH) Liver Transplant Program commenced in 1993, as a continuation of the pioneering program in Linkou CGMH in 1984, we have performed a total of 94 liver transplants for pediatric and adult recipients, 57 of which were with grafts from living donors. Forty-eight of the LDLTs were left-side grafts and nine were right-side grafts. Donor hepatectomies were performed with minimal blood loss and no blood transfusions, which led to prompt recovery and eliminated the risk of transfusion-related disease. Multiple and smaller caliber vessels or ducts are major technical challenges in LDLT. Twelve grafts (21%) had multiple hepatic veins, 22 (39%) had multiple hepatic arteries, and 19 (33%) had multiple bile ducts. Significant technical complications included two hepatic outflow problems, four portal vein problems, and six biliary problems. There was no hospital mortality, but one patient developed septic shock after a radiological procedure and died 4 months after the transplant. The actual patient and graft survival rates were 98.2%. Careful patient selection, judicious preoperative evaluation, meticulous surgical techniques, and prompt detection and management of complications all contribute to optimizing outcomes in LDLT.

Key words. Liver, Liver transplantation, Living-donor liver transplantation, Hepatic vein reconstruction, Biliary complications

Department of Surgery and Liver Transplant Program, Chang Gung University, Chang Gung Memorial Hospital, Kaohsiung Medical Center, 123 Ta-Pei Road, Niao-Sung, Kaohsiung 83305, Taiwan

Introduction

The first liver transplantation in Taiwan was performed in a patient in a life-threatening emergency on March 22, 1984, when a legal definition of brain death had not yet been approved [1]. The successful outcome silenced the medical skeptics, and after extensive discussion and debate, a consensus on brain death was reached in the medical community 7 months after the first liver transplant. Three years later, the Human Organ Transplant Act was passed by Congress and officially proclaimed by the president in 1987. The concept of brain death was then legally defined and accepted [2], paving the way for the subsequent development of pancreas, heart, and lung transplantation. In Taiwan, a total of 229 liver transplants were performed from 1984 until December 31, 2000. One hundred fifty-nine (69.4%) of them were performed at Chang Gung Memorial Hospitals (CGMH). Of living-donor liver transplantations (LDLT) alone, 85% were performed at the CGMH in Kaohsiung (Table 1). Like most countries in Asia, cadaveric organ donation in Taiwan has not increased significantly over the past few years, and LDLT is increasingly resorted to (Fig. 1). The Kaohsiung CGMH program started with LDLT in pediatric patients and expanded to adults using right-lobe grafts in 1999. With greater patient accrual paralleled by growing expertise from accumulated experience, liver transplantation activity at the Kaohsiung CGMH has been increasing steadily over the past few years.

TABLE 1. Liver transplantation in Taiwan (March 1984–December 2000)

Institution	Full-size	Reduced size	Split	Living donor	Total
Kaohsiung Chang Gung Memorial Hospital	38	4	6	57	105
Linkou Chang Gung Memorial Hospital	54	0	0	0	54
National Taiwan University Hospital	30	4	1	10	45
Taipei Veterans General Hospital	13	0	1	0	14
Taichung Veterans General Hospital	2	4	0	0	6
Kaohsiung Medical University Hospital	3	0	0	0	3
Hualien Buddhist Tzu Chi General Hospital	1	0	1	0	2
Total	141	12	9	67	229

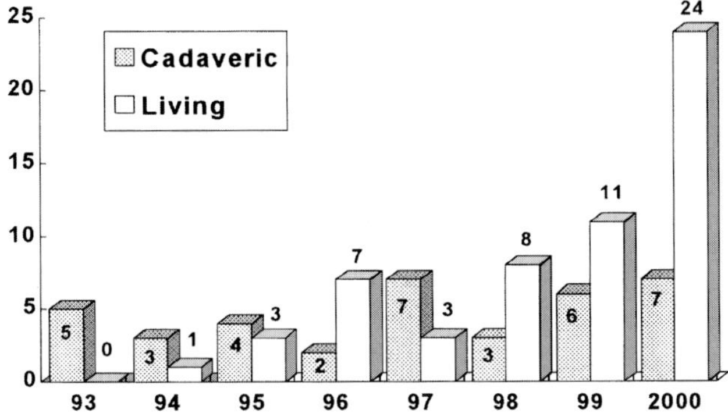

FIG. 1. Annual liver transplantation activity at the Chang Gung Memorial Hospital in Kaohsiung

Patients and Methods

Fifty-seven consecutive cases of LDLT were performed at the CGMH in Kaohsiung, Taiwan, from June 1994 to December 2000. Forty-eight of these LDLTs were left-side grafts and nine were right-side grafts. The donors included 32 mothers, 14 fathers, 4 sons, 3 wives, 2 grandmothers, 1 aunt, and 1 husband. The indications for transplantation were biliary atresia in 40 cases, glycogen storage in 5, primary biliary cirrhosis in 3, hepatitis B virus-related cirrhosis in 3, neonatal hepatitis in 2, hepatitis C virus-related cirrhosis in 2, and 1 case each of Wilson's disease and Alagille syndrome.

Eligible donor volunteers underwent procedures for detailed hepatic vascular and biliary imaging. Doppler ultrasound (US) was used for the initial screening. Magnetic resonance venography (MRV) with angular reconstruction was used to evaluate the hepatic and portal venous anatomy [3]. A computed tomography (CT) scan was used for measurement of graft volume and fat content [4]. Three-dimensional helical computed tomographic cholangiography (3-DCTC) was used to delineate the biliary anatomy [5] until the dye used was phased out in Taiwan. 3-DCTC was replaced by magnetic resonance cholangiography (MRC) from case 21, and intraoperative cholangiography was performed in selected cases. Hepatic angiography was routinely performed to delineate the arterial anatomy, until it was recently replaced with magnetic resonance angiography (MRA) or computed tomographic angiography (CTA). For the recipients, Doppler US, MRV, and MRA were used to confirm the patency of the hepatic artery, and portal and hepatic veins, and to rule out the presence of vascular anomalies, especially in children with biliary atresia.

The type and size of liver grafts obtained was based on an adequate graft-to-recipient weight ratio (GRWR) [6], or the graft volume-to-standard liver volume of the recipient [7], and a minimum of 0.8% or 40%, respectively, was considered acceptable. Donor hepatectomy was carried out without inflow or outflow occlusion according to a technique that has been described previously [8]. After procurement, the graft was weighed and the hepatic vein was carefully inspected. If two or more orifices were found in a left-side graft, one of three techniques of venoplasty was performed to fashion a single wide outflow orifice [9].

Recipient hepatectomy was performed leaving the inferior vena cava (IVC) intact. In children requiring left-side grafts, a triple hepatic venoplasty, consisting of right, middle, and left hepatic veins, was performed to create an adequate outflow orifice. In some older children, a double hepatic venoplasty consisting of the middle and left hepatic veins was used. For right-lobe grafts, the recipient right hepatic vein was widened by excising the IVC wall distally. The graft hepatic vein was anastomosed end-to-end to the recipient hepatic venoplasty. An end-to-end portal vein reconstruction was performed, often using a branch patch of the recipient portal vein in pediatric cases. The hepatic artery was anastomosed using microsurgical techniques. The hepatic duct was anastomosed to the Roux-en-Y limb of the jejunum without a stent, except in tiny ducts of less than 2 mm. Triple-drug immunosuppression with cyclosporine, azathioprine, and steroids was used in all patients. Acute rejection episodes, defined as the presence of typical histological features in association with impaired liver function tests, were treated with pulsed steroids. Tacrolimus was reserved for steroid-resistant rejection or poor bioavailability of cyclosporine.

Results

No complications occurred as a result of the detailed preoperative imaging studies. The mean donor age was 32.8 ± 6.7 years (range 22–53 years), with a mean body weight of 60.1 ± 10.3 kg (range 34–89 kg).

The types of hepatectomy performed included a left lateral segmentectomy (LLS) in 21 cases, extended left lateral segmentectomy (ELLS) in 24 cases, extended left lobectomy (ELL) in 3 cases, extended right lobectomy (ERL) in 4 cases, and right lobectomy (RL) in 5 cases. An ELLS graft consisted of segments II, III, and part of segment IV. ERL or ELL grafts included the middle hepatic vein. The five right-lobe grafts did not include the middle hepatic vein. The mean graft weight was 353.8 ± 173.9 g (range 172–858 g), whereas the mean graft recipient weight ratio was $2.3\% \pm 1.0\%$ (range 0.8%–5.1%). The intraoperative blood loss measured before dividing the hepatic vein

TABLE 2. Comparison of donor outcomes according to type of hepatectomy

Parameter	Left side ($n = 48$)	Right side ($n = 9$)	P value[a]
Operative			
Mean CVP during transection (cmH$_2$0)	7.9 ± 2.5	7.5 ± 2.3	0.801
Operation time (min)	520.6 ± 79.9	625.8 ± 109.5	0.003
Transection time (min)	135.9 ± 51.7	171.8 ± 41.9	0.011
GRWR (%)	2.5 ± 0.9	1.2 ± 0.3	0.000
Blood loss (ml)	62.0 ± 49.3	113.3 ± 97.7	0.019
Postoperative			
Peak AST (U/L)	253.9 ± 123.6	276.9 ± 128.1	0.437
Peak ALT (U/L)	327.4 ± 197.9	263.9 ± 123.4	0.599
Peak TB (U/L)	1.4 ± 0.7	3.9 ± 2.3	0.000
Peak creatinine (mg%)	0.8 ± 0.2	0.9 ± 0.1	0.152

CVP, central venous pressure; GRWR, graft–recipient body weight ratio; AST, aspartate aminotransferase; ALT, alanine aminotransferase; TB, total bilirubin
[a] Calculated using the Mann–Whitney U test
All data are given as mean ± standard deviation

ranged from 15 to 360 ml, with a mean of 70.1 ± 61.3 ml (median 60 ml). No blood, fresh-frozen plasma, albumin, or any other blood derivatives were transfused in any donors intraoperatively or during the postoperative period. A comparison of donor characteristics, and intraoperative and postoperative parameters according to type of hepatectomy are shown in Table 2. The immediate postoperative course in the 57 donors was uneventful. All donors were discharged between 5 and 17 days after surgery (mean 7 days). Two donors (donors 39 and 45) required prolonged hospitalization because of exacerbation of a duodenal ulcer. Three donors were readmitted; one (donor 17) for gastroenteritis, which required only conservative treatment, and the other two (donors 21 and 43) for a biloma at the cut edge of the remnant liver. These were successfully treated by percutaneous drainage. None of the donors required any further surgery. Currently, all donors are completely healthy with normal liver function, and have resumed their predonation levels of activity. Four of the maternal donors subsequently gave birth to normal babies 2–4 years after surgery. The anatomic variants in the 57 grafts included 12 (21%) who had multiple hepatic veins requiring venoplasty, 22 (39%) who had multiple hepatic arteries, and 19 (33%) who had multiple bile ducts.

In the recipients, the mean age was 10.0 ± 16.1 years (range 0.6–56 years), with a mean body weight of 20.5 ± 19.5 kg (range 5.1–86 kg). Fourteen patients (24.6%) experienced a total of 18 episodes of histologically proven acute cellular rejection; 12 occurred within the first posttransplant month and 6 after. All responded to steroid pulse therapy and there were no cases of steroid resistance or chronic rejection. However, two patients were changed to tacrolimus because of the poor bioavailability of cyclosporine.

Technical complications included two hepatic vein stenoses, four acute portal vein occlusions, and six biliary problems, including a missed biliary radicle, multiple intrahepatic duct strictures, bile leak from the Roux limb of the hepaticojejunostomy, repeated cholangitis related to biliary stenting, and two anastomotic bile leaks. Three of these six cases required surgical management, including reanastomosis of the missed bile duct, evacuation of a biloma with septic manifestations, and removal of a retained biliary stent. Other significant recipient morbidities that required relaparotomies included intraabdominal hemorrhage ($n = 2$), bowel perforation ($n = 2$), a fragmented Jackson-Pratt drain ($n = 1$), removal of an abdominal wall prosthesis ($n = 1$), and late bowel obstruction ($n = 2$). There was no documented hepatic artery thrombosis in this series. There was no hospital mortality, although one patient (case 48) developed septic shock after a radiological procedure and died 4 months after the transplant. At a mean follow-up of 2.3 ± 1.8 years (range 0.3–6.9 years), actual patient and graft survival rates are both 98%.

Discussion

Obtaining grafts from live donors for liver transplantation is an important resource in countries where cadaveric donation is rare. This is currently the only way of effectively increasing the liver graft supply in Asia. While it was initially established to provide grafts for pediatric recipients, the development of techniques for right-lobe liver grafting have expanded the indications to include adult recipients. The majority of LDLTs in Taiwan are performed at the Kaohsiung CGMH, which is fast becoming a major referral center for the whole country, with 39% of recipients coming from northern Taiwan, 33% from central Taiwan, and 28% from southern Taiwan. As the public is becoming more aware of LDLT, patients often come with volunteer liver donors. Since adult-to-adult LDLT was started in our institution, donors have included spouses and children. An important limiting factor in our setting is obtaining prior approval from the National Health Insurance Bureau, which is a requirement in Taiwan if the patient is to take advantage of this form of payment.

The donor operation should be carefully planned based on accurate preoperative imaging studies, and performed with the least possible risk to the volunteer. As imaging techniques improve and available modalities are better utilized, the surgeons are provided with the adequate "road-map" that is necessary to determine the extent of the hepatectomy required. We aim to avoid blood transfusion and minimize blood loss by employing meticulous dissection and careful transection of the liver parenchyma [8]. In this series of 57 donor hepatectomies we have never had the occasion to transfuse blood products, and thus the risk of contracting a transfusion-related disease is eliminated. A comparison of outcomes between right-lobe and left-lobe graft donors showed that the operation time, transection time, and blood loss for right-lobe hepatectomy were higher, although postoperative recovery in the two groups was equally good (see Table 2). Peak total bilirubin was significantly higher after right donor lobectomy, although serial determinations showed a return to normal within 7–10 postoperative days (data not shown). Biliary complications occur in about 4% of living liver donors [10], and the incidence in the series reported here is 3.5% (2/57). The medical complications were few, and were resolved with conservative treatment.

Segmental liver transplantation is particularly challenging because of the issues of size matching and smaller caliber vessels and ducts. Extremes of size mismatch are equally detrimental to graft function [6]. In our series, GRWR was within the acceptable minimum, while two babies with large-for-size grafts required Goretex prostheses for abdominal closure. Pediatric patients are at risk of having large-for-size grafts, while for adults, small-for-size grafts can be circumvented by taking an extended right-lobe graft including the middle hepatic vein [11], which we did in four of our cases. The reconstruction of small-caliber and/or multiple vessels or ducts is a major technical hurdle in segmental liver transplantation. The left-side hepatic venous anatomy tends to be more varied, and separate left superior or marginal veins are not uncommon. We have opted to do a single outflow reconstruction whenever possible, by performing venoplasty of the graft hepatic veins to form a single outflow orifice. This is matched with a triple venoplasty in the recipient, which results in a single, short outflow trunk that is less prone to twisting or kinking [9].

In this series there were only two significant outflow problems that were due to stenoses at the anastomotic site and were managed by the placement of vascular stents. In two cases that had segment-3 veins draining into the middle hepatic vein at a distance from the segment-2 hepatic vein, the distal middle hepatic vein of the donor was taken with the graft to obtain a single outflow orifice in the graft. This technique is useful to avoid multiple anastomoses in the recipient, and was previously described by Tojimbara et al. [12].

Inflow reconstruction is basically more simple and straightforward than outflow reconstruction. For portal vein anastomoses we routinely use a branch patch in the pediatric recipient unless the main portal vein is of adequate size. The ligation of collaterals often helps to improve portal inflow. In four cases, low or absent flow was detected intraoperatively and was managed by immediate revision of the anastomosis with or without a thrombectomy. For arterial reconstruction in grafts with multiple hepatic arteries, the bigger one was anastomosed first, and if there was good backflow from the remaining one(s), then they were simply ligated [13]. In this series there has been no documented arterial thombosis, although we used urokinase infusion in two patients who had decreased arterial flow with an accompanying derangement in liver function in the postoperative period.

The reconstruction of multiple bile ducts, which tend to be tiny, may be difficult. In this series, biliary complications occurred at an incidence of 10% (6/57), and half of them were in patients who had multiple small-caliber hepatic ducts. Two of them developed bilomas from an anastomotic leak, while one had repeated episodes of cholangitis that could have been due to a retained biliary stent. This particular patient (case 47) improved after surgical removal of the biliary stent. It is therefore important to obtain a single bile duct orifice in the graft in order to avoid dealing with tiny ducts that may be difficult to reconstruct.

LDLT is a technically demanding operation that can now be performed with a reasonably high rate of success. Donor safety is of primary concern, and should not be compromised at any cost. Careful donor and recipient selection will allow graft–recipient size requirements to be met, and surgical expertise will allow for innovations or adjustments in technique to accommodate acceptable anatomic variants. The long-term outcomes of LDLT remain to be seen, and will eventually reinforce the rationale for this type of operation. In the meantime it will continue to be an important source of liver grafts until more sophisticated alternatives to treat end-stage liver disease become clinically applicable.

References

1. Chen CL, Wang KL, Lee MC, et al. (1987) Liver transplantation for Wilson's disease. Report of the first successful liver transplant in Taiwan. Jpn J Transplant 22:178–184
2. Chen CL, Wang KL, Hui YL, et al. (1992) Liver transplantation in Taiwan: the Chang Gung experience. Cancer Chemother Pharmacol 31:S162–S165
3. Cheng YF, Chen CL, Huang TL, et al. (1999) Magnetic resonance of the hepatic veins with angular reconstruction: application in living related liver transplantation. Transplantation 68:267–271
4. Cheng YF, Chen CL, Lai CY, et al. (2001) Radiological assessment of fatty liver in liver transplantation. Transplantation 71:1221–1225
5. Cheng YF, Lee TY, Chen CL, et al. (1997) Three-dimensional helical computed tomographic cholangiography application to living related hepatic transplantation. Clin Transplant 11:209–213
6. Kiuchi T, Kasahara M, Uryuhara K, et al. (1999) Impact of graft size mismatching on graft prognosis in liver transplantation from living donors. Transplantation 67:321–327
7. Lo CM, Fan ST, Liu CL, et al. (1999) Minimum graft size for successful living donor liver transplantation. Transplantation 68:1112–1116

8. Chen CL, Chen YS, de Villa VH, et al. (2000) Minimal blood loss living donor hepatectomy. Transplantation 69:2580–2586
9. de Villa VH, Chen CL, Chen YS, et al. (2000) Outflow tract reconstruction in living donor liver transplantation. Transplantation 70:1604–1608
10. Marcos A (2000) Right-lobe living donor liver transplantation. Liver Transplant 6 (S2):S59–S63
11. Lo CM, Fan ST, Liu CL, et al. (1997) Adult-to-adult living donor liver transplantation using extended right-lobe grafts. Ann Surg 226:261
12. Tojimbara T, Fuchinoue S, Nakajima I, et al. (1998) Analysis of post-operative liver function of donors in living-related liver transplantation. Transplantation 66:1035
13. Furuta S, Ikegami T, Nakazawa Y, et al. (1997) Hepatic artery reconstruction in living donor liver transplantation from the microsurgeon's point of view. Liver Transplant Surg 3:388–393

Impact of Small-for-Size Graft on Graft Surgical and Postoperative Complications in Adult Living Donor Liver Transplantation

Koichi Tanaka

The adequacy of the size of the liver is the major limitation and most critical issue associated with adult living donor liver transplantation (LDLT). The impact of graft size on the outcome of the transplantion patient is clearly demonstrated in our 1-year survival results in non-intensive care unit (ICU)-bound patients. The 1-year survival rate was 91.8% in those with a graft/recipient weight ratio (GRWR) of ≥1.0%, 79.5% among those with a GRWR of 0.8%–1.0%, and 59.7% among those with a GRWR of <0.8%. The difference by graft size was even greater in ICU-bound patients. The decreased survival in small-for-size grafts was accompanied by poor early graft function and hepatocyte injury as well as by prolonged cholestasis. Moreover, the incidence of surgical complications (e.g., hemorrhage, intestinal perforation) and septic complications were in inverse correlation with graft size relative to the recipient. The posttransplant serum creatinine level is inversely correlated with graft size; and the incidence of bacteremia within 1 month after transplantation increased as the GRWR decreased. With technical refinements backed by precise knowledge of anatomical variations and physiology, we believe right lobe LDLT has become a highly effective treatment modality, with acceptable risk for both donors and recipients. In countries where cadaveric organ donation is not well organized, this procedure will remain, at least for a while, in the mainstream of liver transplantation. However, we should always bear in mind that adult LDLT is still at an early stage and must continue to undergo critical review.

Department of Transplantation Immunology, Kyoto University Graduate School of Medicine, Kyoto, Japan

Living-Donor Liver Transplantation Using Left-Liver Graft and Hepatic Vein Reconstruction

Masatoshi Makuuchi and Yasuhiko Sugawara

Summary. Several new methods have been developed to make living-donor liver transplantation safer. We describe our techniques in hepatic vein reconstruction. Taking the left liver with a caudate lobe graft is useful to overcome the problems of a small graft. Hepatic vein reconstruction appears necessary to allow proportional regeneration of the caudate lobe. A right-liver graft without a middle hepatic vein trunk is another option in this situation. Unless intrahepatic venous communication can be seen in the right-liver, the reconstruction of middle hepatic vein tributaries is essential to prevent congestion of the right paramedian sector.

Key words. Caudate lobe, Middle hepatic vein, Vein reconstruction

Introduction

Living-donor liver transplantation (LDLT) is now accepted worldwide as an effective modality to save end-stage liver failure patients. To make LDLT safer, several new methods have been developed. We describe our techniques in hepatic vein reconstruction.

Vein Reconstruction in Left-Liver Graft with a Caudate Lobe

A major limitation in adult LDLT is obtaining a graft of adequate size. To overcome this difficulty, the left-liver graft with a caudate lobe was devised. The Spiegel lobe corresponds to only 3%–4% of the total liver volume. However,

Artificial Organ and Transplantation Division, Department of Surgery, The University of Tokyo, 7-3-1 Hongo, Bunkyo-ku, Tokyo 113-8655, Japan

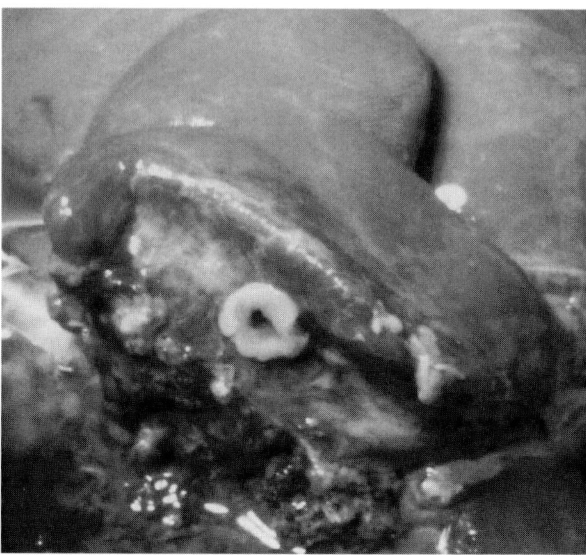

FIG. 1. Stump of a hepatic vein draining the caudate lobe with a cuff of caval wall

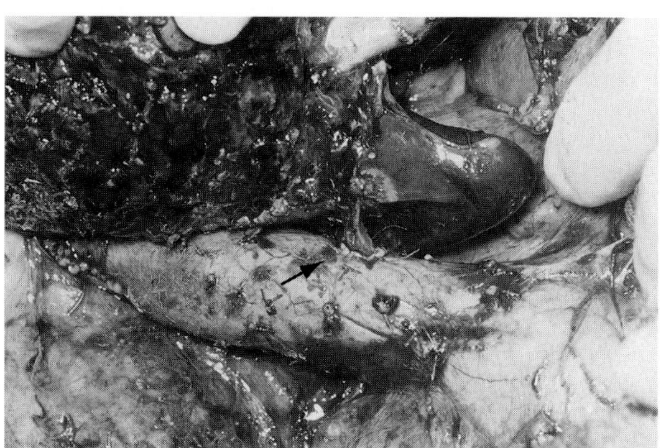

FIG. 2. Reconstruction of the caudate hepatic vein is carried out following reconstruction of the left and middle hepatic veins. *Arrow* indicates anastomosis

in conjunction with a left-liver graft, it provides a gain in weight of 8%–12% [1]. According to the cast study by Couinaud [2], 69% (66/96) of Spiegel lobes had a single vein and 20% had two veins. Most of the veins (91%, 115/126) entered directly into the vena cava. That study indicated that one or two veins of the Spiegel lobe should be reconstructed to prevent venous congestion of the caudate lobe.

The hepatic vein of the caudate lobe can be resected with a cuff of the vena cava, which looks like a Carrel's patch (Fig. 1). In the recipient operation, reconstruction of the caudate hepatic vein is carried out first (Fig. 2). Then the trunk of the left and middle hepatic veins (MHV) of the recipient and the graft are anastomosed.

To estimate the success of the reconstruction of the caudate hepatic vein, computed tomography was performed 1 month after the operation. Regeneration of the left liver and the Spiegel lobe were comparable with that of the left liver. Using the left liver with a caudate lobe, the rate of cholestasis has decreased from 43% (6/14) to 15% (4/26), but this difference is not statistically significant ($P = 0.12$).

Right-Liver Graft

The side of the liver in the donor that should be used as a graft is now a topic of heated debate. A right-liver graft can help to alleviate the problem of graft size disparity in adult LDLT. However, we do not think that right hepatectomy is a sufficiently safe form of donor hepatectomy because the safety of this procedure varies, depending mainly on the volume of the left liver. We do not perform right hepatectomy if the volume of the left liver is estimated to be less than 30% of the total liver.

Hepatic Vein Reconstruction in "Modified" Right-Liver Graft

Fan and co-workers [3] used the right liver with the MHV as a graft. This method is a good approach because the MHV is a major draining vein of the right paramedian sector, and the draining area of segment IV is limited. However, LDLT using an extended right liver graft increases the extent of the donor operation, and can present an important ethical issue [4].

A "modified" right-liver graft without a MHV trunk might avoid this problem. Whether or not the hepatic vein needs reconstruction in this type of graft is still unclear. Kam and co-workers [5] preserved the MHV between the tributaries of segments VIII and V without reconstruction. Tanaka, at Kyoto University, stated that he had had little experience of complications due to severe graft congestion after LDLT using a right-liver graft without the MHV trunk. In the United States and Europe, most liver transplant surgeons do not reconstruct the MHV tributaries [6].

In contrast, Lee et al. [7] raised a different concern. They claimed that a right-liver graft without the MHV trunk could cause severe congestion of the right paramedian sector. This graft congestion can cause severe graft dysfunction and septic complications. They now reconstruct all venous tributaries of the MHV.

Criteria for the Reconstruction of MHV Tributaries

Couinaud and Nogueira [8] reported that intrahepatic hepatic vein communication was recognized in 25 of 30 casts. However, these findings might not reflect normal physiological conditions. Hepatic wedge venography can easily demonstrate the portal venous system [9]. In Budd-Chiari syndrome, the arterial blood flows into the portal vein and is drained via the unobstructed hepatic vein.

Against this background, we agree with Lee's proposal and recently reported tentative criteria for the reconstruction of MHV tributaries [10]. From January to October 2000, we performed 30 LDLTs. When the left liver with the MHV was used as a graft, congestion of the right paramedian sector was evaluated under occlusion of the MHV and right hepatic artery in the donor. Congestion of segment IV in the graft was evaluated by occlusion of the left hepatic artery.

The absolute indications for hepatic vein reconstruction are when the surface of the liver turns dark purple after the division of MHV tributaries. However, none of the grafts in our series satisfied this criterion. Intrahepatic

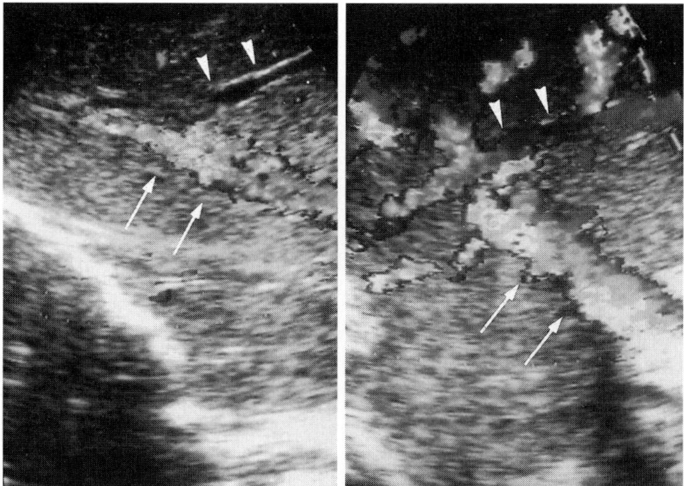

FIG. 3. Left-liver graft without the MHV trunk. After reconstruction of the left hepatic vein and portal vein, Doppler ultrasonography was performed. Blood flow signals were not seen in the middle hepatic vein, and the portal flow was regurgitated (*left*). After reconstruction of a branch of the MHV, normal blood flow signals were obtained in both the hepatic vein and the portal vein in segment 4 (*right*). *Arrows*, portal flow; *arrowheads*, hepatic vein flow

venous communication was seen in six of 30 grafts. In these grafts, intra-operative color Doppler ultrasound revealed many communicating channels between the MHV and inferior right hepatic vein or right hepatic vein after clamping of the MHV. However, in the remaining 24 grafts, when the MHV was clamped, venous flow in the MHV was eliminated and reversed portal flow was recognized in the portal branch (Fig. 3). In these grafts, when the hepatic artery was clamped, a discolored area emerged on the surface of the graft. In such cases, hepatic vein reconstruction seems mandatory.

Conclusions

Hepatic vein reconstruction appears necessary for regeneration of the caudate lobe in proportion to the left liver. When intrahepatic venous communication cannot be seen in the right liver, reconstruction of MHV tributaries is mandatory to prevent graft congestion.

References

1. Takayama T, Makuuchi M, Kubota K, et al. (2000) Living-related transplantation of left liver plus caudate lobe. J Am Coll Surg 190:635–638
2. Couinaud C (1957) Le foie. Etudes anatomiques et chirurgicales. Masson, Paris, pp 187–208
3. Lo CM, Fan ST, Liu CL, et al. (1997) Adult-to-adult living donor liver transplantation using extended right lobe grafts. Ann Surg 226:261–269
4. Sugawara Y, Makuuchi M (1999) Technical advances in living-related liver transplantation. J Hepatobiliary Pancreat Surg 6:245–253
5. Trotter JF, Wachs M, Trouillot T, et al. (2000) Evaluation of 100 patients for living donor liver transplantation. Liver Transplant 6:290–295
6. Marcos A, Fisher RA, Ham JM, et al. (1999) Right lobe living donor liver transplantation. Transplantation 68:798–803
7. Lee SG, Park KM, Hwang S, et al. (1999) Adult-to-adult living donor liver transplantation at the Asian Medical Center, Seoul, Korea. Transplant Proc 31:456–458
8. Couinaud C, Nogueira C (1958) Les veins sus-hepatique chez l'homme. Acta Anat 34: 84–110
9. Rapparport AM (1951) Hepatic venography. Acta Radiol 36:165
10. Sano K, Makuuchi M, Takayama T, et al. (2000) Technical dilemma in living donor or split-liver transplant. Hepatogastroenterology 47:1208–1209

Results of Living-Donor Liver Transplantation in Hong Kong

SHEUNG-TAT FAN, CHUNG-MAU LO, CHI-LEUNG LIU, and WILLIAM IGNACE WEI

Summary. At Queen Mary Hospital, the University of Hong Kong Medical Centre, 88 live-donor liver transplantations were performed between 1993 and 2001. Sixteen children received left lateral segment grafts, one child received a left-lobe graft, five adults received left-lobe grafts, and 66 adults received right-lobe grafts, all from family members or friends. Five children (29%) and 29 adults (40%) were managed in the intensive care unit before liver transplantation. There was no donor mortality. The overall survival rate of the pediatric patients was 75% (12/16). When left-lobe grafts were used in adult patients, the survival rate was 100% (3/3) for those with fulminant hepatic failure, and 0% (2/2) for those with cirrhosis. With the use of right-lobe grafts, the overall survival rate was 83% (55/66). There was no difference in the long-term survival of patients undergoing elective or emergency transplantation.

Key words. Live donor, Liver transplantation, Right-lobe graft

Introduction

The first two live-donor liver transplantations (LDLT) in the world were performed by Raia et al. in Brazil in 1989 [1]. Both donors donated the left lateral segments and were well after the operation, but the two pediatric recipients died after the operation. In 1989, Strong et al. [2] performed the first successful LDLT in a child using a left lateral segment graft from her mother. Thereafter, the LDLT program for pediatric patients has proliferated rapidly

Centre for the Study of Liver Disease and Department of Surgery, University of Hong Kong Medical Centre, Queen Mary Hospital, 102 Pokfulam Road, Hong Kong

in many parts of the world, particularly in Japan, where cadaveric organ donation was prohibited before 1997.

The application of LDLT to adult recipients was initiated by Haberal et al. in 1992, but the attempts were not successful [3]. In 1993, Makuuchi and co-workers had the first success when they transplanted the left lobe from a 25-year-old man to his 53-year-old mother [4]. In 1994, the authors performed a similar operation between a 59-kg woman suffering from fulminant hepatic failure and her 82-kg husband [5]. In such a situation, when the donor is heavier than the recipient, the left-lobe graft volume is sufficient to support the metabolic functions of the patient. When the donor and the recipient are of similar body size, the volume of the left lobe is insufficient; when the recipient has preexisting portal hypertension, the graft may sustain serious injury and primary graft nonfunction results. To extend the application of LDLT to all adult recipients, the authors initiated a technique using an extended right-lobe graft in 1996 [6]. In this chapter, we give a detailed account of LDLT at the University of Hong Kong Medical Centre, Queen Mary Hospital, Hong Kong.

Patients and Methods

From October 1993 to February 2001, LDLT was performed in 17 children and 71 adults at the University of Hong Kong Medical Centre, Queen Mary Hospital, Hong Kong. The indications for LDLT are listed in Table 1. The median age of the children was 1.2 years (range 0.5–11 years), while that of the adults was 46 years (range 17–68 years). Five children (29%) and 29 adults (40%) were managed in the intensive care unit before liver transplantation. The relationships between the donors and the patients are listed in Table 2. Left lateral segment grafts were used in 16 children; left-lobe grafts were used in

TABLE 1. Indications for live-donor liver transplantation

	Children ($n = 17$)	Adults ($n = 71$)
Hepatitis B cirrhosis	0	32
Primary biliary cirrhosis	0	2
Secondary biliary cirrhosis	0	1
Fulminant hepatic failure	4	13
Acute-on-chronic hepatitis B	0	21
Biliary atresia	10	0
Alagille syndrome	1	0
Ruptured adenoma	0	1
Autoimmune hepatitis	0	1
Graft rejection	1	0
Graft hepatitis	1	0

TABLE 2. Donor relationships

	Children ($n = 17$)	Adults ($n = 71$)
Spouse	0	28
Parent	14	4
Brother/sister	1	12
Son/daughter	0	18
Brother/sister-in-law	0	3
Son-in-law	0	1
Uncle/aunt	1	2
Friend	1	2
Nephew	0	1

one child and five adults; and right-lobe grafts were used in 66 adults. The left-lobe grafts were used in the first five adult-to-adult LDLTs. After failure in two patients, right-lobe grafts were used exclusively in all subsequent patients.

Donor Evaluation

All donors were evaluated preoperatively by hematology, biochemistry, and virus serology tests, and by a clinical psychologist to ensure that the donation was truly voluntary. Computed tomography was performed to delineate the hepatic vein anatomy and volumetry. The donor was accepted if the laboratory test results were normal and the donated liver volume measured more than 40% of the estimated standard liver volume of the recipient [7]. A right-lobe donor must have a remnant left-lobe volume which is more than 30% of the total volume before acceptance [8]. Hepatic arteriography was then performed to delineate the hepatic artery and portal vein anatomy. The origin of the left medial segment hepatic artery was carefully studied and noted before the donor operation to avoid accidental damage during the donor operation. The length of the right portal vein and its anomalies were studied.

The donors were prepared with great care on the operating table to avoid sores at the pressure points. All donors had undergone measures against deep vein thrombosis. Heparin was given to two female donors who had a history of taking oral contraceptive pills.

Right-Lobe Graft Donor Operation

The laparotomy was performed via bilateral subcostal incisions with an upward midline extension. Intraoperative ultrasonography was performed to identify the configuration of the middle hepatic vein anatomy, and in particular its relationship with the left hepatic vein and the inferior vena cava. The presence of the hepatic vein of the cranial portion of the left medial segment

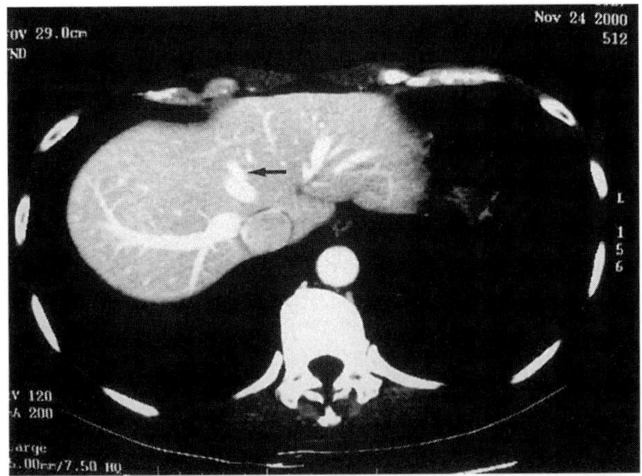

FIG. 1. Computed tomography scan showing the hepatic vein anatomy. The *arrow* indicates segment 4b draining into the middle hepatic vein. The branch could be preserved to avoid venous congestion of segment 4 in the donor

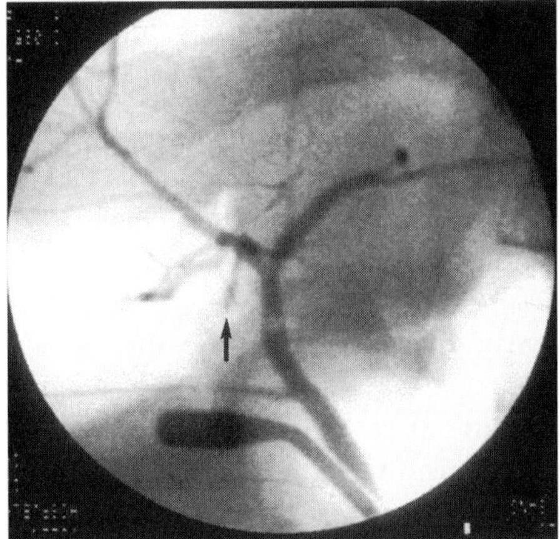

FIG. 2. Cholangiogram showing the biliary anatomy. The bulldog vascular clamp allows complete filling of the intrahepatic duct. The metal clip placed over the right hepatic duct marks the site of division of the duct (*arrow*)

(segment 4b) (Fig. 1) was examined, and if present, it was protected and retained in the left-lobe remnant. The presence of a large inferior right hepatic vein (draining segment 6) or middle right hepatic vein (draining segment 7) was also checked, and preserved for the graft if present. Operative cholangiography was performed by cannulation of the cystic duct, using undiluted radiographic contrast and under fluoroscopy. We prefer fluoroscopy because it allows real-time visualization of the sequence of filling the intrahepatic duct with radiographic contrast medium. The right posterior segment of the hepatic duct is the most dependent and was therefore filled first, while the left lateral and medial segments of the hepatic ducts which are located at a more dorsal position were filled last. A small bulldog vascular clamp was applied across the supraduodenal part of the common bile duct for retrograde filling of the intrahepatic duct with contrast medium (Fig. 2).

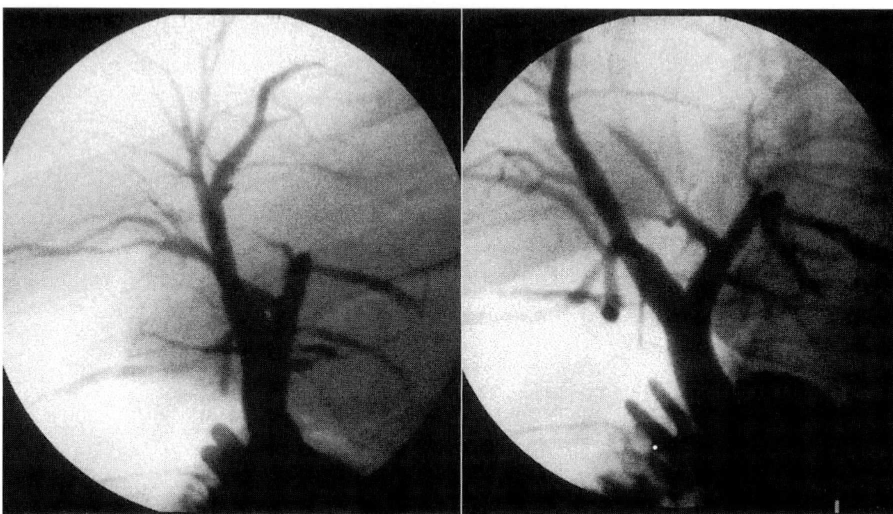

FIG. 3. Cholangiogram obtained in the posteroanterior position (*left*) is difficult to interpret as the liver has rotated into the right subphrenic cavity because the donor is relatively old. Rotation of the X-ray tube toward the right side of the donor shows the anatomy of the biliary tract clearly (*right*). There were two right hepatic ducts, with the right posterior hepatic duct joining the left duct

By rotating the X-ray tube, the correct orientation and recognition of the left and right hepatic ducts could be performed (Fig. 3). Before cholangiography, a gentle dissection at the liver hilum was made to identify the confluence of the left and right hepatic ducts. A large Liga clip was applied to the proposed site of division of the right hepatic duct. The site of division was verified on the cholangiogram (Fig. 2). Diathermy coagulation was then applied to the liver capsule just above the site of the proposed right hepatic duct division. This point was the lowest point of the liver parenchyma division on the inferior surface of the liver (Fig. 4). A hilar dissection was made to isolate the right hepatic artery and the right portal vein. Dissection of the right hepatic artery was limited to the right side of the common bile duct and was not made in the space between the right hepatic duct and right hepatic artery beyond the proposed line of division of the right hepatic duct. This is essential to avoid ischemic damage to the right hepatic duct and common bile duct. Several caudate lobe portal vein branches were ligated and divided to allow sufficient length of the right portal vein for the harvesting procedure. The right lobe of the liver was then rotated toward the left side for division of the right triangular ligament and tiny venous branches between the anterior surface of the inferior vena cava and the posterior surface of the paracaval portion of the caudate lobe. The liver rotation was intermittent to avoid pro-

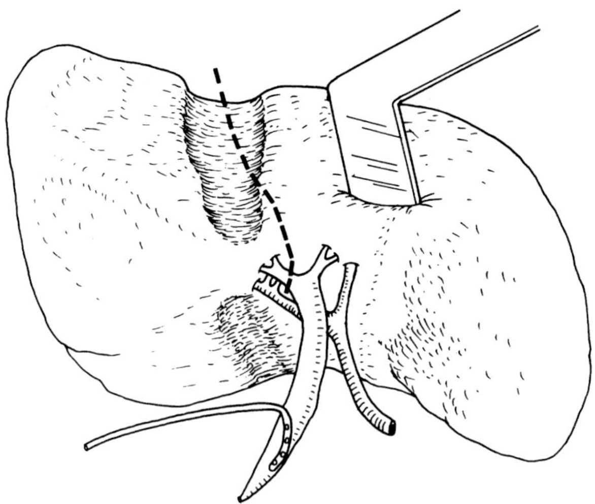

Fig. 4. Schematic diagram showing the line of liver transection at the inferior surface of the liver. The line should deviate to the left side of the gallbladder fossa and stop at the point of the proposed site of the right hepatic division, which is determined by operative cholangiography

longed twisting of the inflow and outflow vascular pedicles of the left lobe. All gauzes and packs were removed from the liver hilum to allow space for rotation and prevent compression of the portal vein. The right hepatic vein and inferior or middle right hepatic vein larger than 5 mm were preserved until the time of harvesting.

The liver was transected at a plane just to the left side of the middle hepatic vein using an ultrasonic dissector. The transection plane was demarcated on the liver surface by temporary occlusion of the right hepatic artery and right portal vein. In case the demarcation was not obvious, the transection plane was verified by intraoperative ultrasonography. The plane at which the middle hepatic vein could be seen with the inferior vena cava was the correct plane [7]. During liver transection, neither inflow nor outflow vascular occlusion was employed. When the liver transection approached the hilum, the right hepatic duct together with Glisson's sheath was encircled and divided at the site determined by operative cholangiography [7]. Brisk bleeding from the divided duct was encountered and controlled by pressure and suturing using 6-0 prolene. Careful inspection was made to identify the number of right hepatic duct branches and any duct missed by cholangiography. The divided ends at the confluence of the hepatic ducts were closed transversely by a continuous 5-0 polydioxanone monofilament absorbable suture. The liver transection was continued down to the caudate lobe and the junction of the middle hepatic vein with the left hepatic vein or inferior vena cava. Lifting the paracaval portion of the caudate lobe with the assistant's index finger or an instrument facilitated the transection process.

At the time of harvesting, the right portal vein was clamped and cannulated with a catheter that was connected to cold Hartman solution. In case the right portal vein was short, two cannulae were inserted into the two branches of the portal vein via a single opening in the anterior surface of the right portal vein. The right hepatic artery was clamped and divided. The hepatic vein was clamped using vascular staplers and divided on the graft side. Blood that escaped from the graft was recovered and collected in a red cell saver for the first 20 donors, but not for subsequent donors. The stumps of the right hepatic artery and right portal vein were closed by continuous prolene sutures. Methylene blue was injected into the common bile duct via the cystic duct cannula to detect bile leakage from the right hepatic duct stump and transection surface. Operative cholangiography was repeated to reaffirm the integrity of the biliary tract. Intraoperative ultrasonography was repeated to confirm that there was no blood vessel injury. The falciform ligament was sutured to the anterior abdominal wall to prevent rotation of the left lobe into the right subphrenic cavity. An abdominal drain was not used.

Left-Lobe Graft Donor Operation

The operation was similar to right-lobe donation except that the left portal structures were freed and the middle hepatic vein was included in the left-lobe graft. The caudate lobe was not included in the graft.

Left Lateral Segment Graft Donor Operation

The operation was similar to left-lobe graft donation except that the liver transection was made on the right side of the falciform ligament. The left medial segment portal vein and the hepatic artery were divided and ligated at the transection plane. If the left medial segment hepatic artery ran into the right side of the umbilical fissura, it was preserved and served to maintain the viability of the left medial segment.

Right-Lobe Graft Recipient Operation

The laparotomy was performed via bilateral subcostal incisions with an upward midline incision. A hilar dissection was made to free the cystic duct, common hepatic duct (which was divided and ligated), and two or three branches of the hepatic artery. Microvascular clamps were used to control the hepatic artery branches, and the distal sides were clamped and divided with a scalpel to reduce intimal injury. The portal vein and its two branches were freed. The liver was then mobilized by dividing the left and right triangular ligaments, venous branches between the anterior surface of the inferior vena cava, and the posterior surface of the caudate lobe until the right hepatic vein and the common trunk of the middle and left hepatic veins were isolated. When the right-lobe graft was available, the portal vein was clamped and its two branches were divided, and the right hepatic vein and the common trunk of the middle and left hepatic veins were clamped. The right hepatic vein was divided near the liver, while the liver parenchyma 2–3 cm proximal to the common trunk of the middle and left hepatic veins was incised to allow sufficient length of the middle or left hepatic vein for anastomosis. The liver parenchyma surrounding the middle and left hepatic veins was removed and tiny venous openings were sutured individually. A small vascular clamp was applied to the edge of the middle or left hepatic vein and the original vascular clamp was released to check for holes in the other hepatic vein, which were secured by fine sutures. The inferior vena cava was mobilized from the retroperitoneum. Complete hemostasis was achieved before implantation. No veno-venous bypass was used in the 37 most recent patients.

The inferior vena cava was cross-clamped in preparation for hepatic vein reconstruction. The hepatic vein orifices were measured and compared with the corresponding orifices of the liver graft. In cases where the right hepatic vein orifice of the right-lobe graft was larger than that of the recipient, the inferior vena cava was slit open to a size that matched the graft. In cases where the middle hepatic vein orifice of the recipient was smaller than that of the graft, the left hepatic vein was chosen if it was larger in size, or the septum between the middle and left hepatic veins was divided to create a large opening for anastomosis.

The right hepatic vein anastomosis was reconstructed by running 3-0 prolene sutures, and was made as short and wide as possible. For the middle hepatic vein anastomosis, the aim was to create a large opening without tension or twisting. A growth factor of 1.0 cm was allowed at the time of knotting to prevent constriction of the anastomosis. The orifice of the right portal vein of the graft was measured and compared with that of the left or right portal vein of the recipient. Matched portal vein branches were used for anastomosis. Hepatic artery anastomosis was performed by a microvascular surgery technique. Bilioenteric anastomosis was performed in all patients except the last three. An internal stent was used to splint the bilioenteric anastomosis. In the first 30 patients, only a small opening was made in the jejunum because we were afraid of creating a bowel opening of excessive size on subsequent manipulation. After realizing that a jejunum opening smaller than the size of the right hepatic duct orifice was a possible cause of anastomotic stenosis and leakage, we adopted a routine of making an opening that was by the same size as the right hepatic duct orifice to achieve a size-matched anastomosis. In cases where these were two right hepatic duct orifices that required two separated bilioenteric anastomoses, the two jejunal openings were made at a distance of about three times the distance between the two right hepatic duct orifices. This was necessary because the jejunum tended to contract after the openings were made, and if sufficient distance between the two orifices was not provided, there would not be enough jejunal wall to suture the anastomoses. In the last three recipients, a duct-to-duct anastomosis was made. No internal or external stent was used in these three recipients.

Left-Lobe Graft Recipient Operation

The hepatectomy procedure was the same as the right-lobe operation. Implantation started with side-clamping of the middle and left hepatic veins and part of the inferior vena cava. The septum between the middle and left hepatic veins was divided, and the right wall of the middle hepatic vein was divided into the lumen of the inferior vena cava so that a large opening was created for subsequent anastomosis. The portal vein, hepatic artery, and bilioenteric anastomoses were reconstructed in the same manner as in the right-lobe graft. The falciform ligament was anchored to the anterior abdominal wall to prevent graft rotation into the right subphrenic cavity and kinking of the left portal vein.

Left Lateral Segment Recipient Operation

The operation was similar to that of left-lobe graft operation. The main difficulty encountered was in the portal vein anastomosis because the portal vein in biliary atresia patients was atretic. In this situation, the left and right portal veins were dissected and trimmed to a size that matched the left portal vein of the graft. The posterior layer of the portal vein anastomosis was reconstructed by running 6-0 polydioxanone monofilament absorbable suture, while interrupted sutures were used in the anterior layer for the most recent patients. During hepatic artery and bilioenteric anastomoses, packs were placed in the right subphrenic cavity to prevent graft rotation and kinking of the left portal vein. Before closure of the abdominal wound, the falciform ligament was sutured to the abdominal wall.

Postoperative Care of Donors

The donors were cared for in the intensive care unit with special attention to adequate tissue oxygenation and perfusion. They were given adequate analgesics and intravenous fluids. The central venous pressure was maintained at a low level to avoid congestion of the liver remnant. The central venous catheter was removed on postoperative day 1 to eliminate the chance of catheter-related infection. Chest physiotherapy and incentive spirometry were routinely given.

Postoperative Care of the Recipients

The recipients were cared for in the intensive care unit with special attention to adequate tissue oxygenation, perfusion, sedation, mechanical ventilation, and monitoring of their coagulation profile and drain output. Mechanical ventilation ceased on postoperative day 1 if the graft function was satisfactory. Drain output was replaced by fresh frozen plasma if the international normalized ratio (INR) exceeded 1.8, and by plasma if the INR was less than 1.8. The immunosuppression protocol consisted of a steroid and FK506. FK506 was started at a dosage of 0.15 mg per kg per day (divided into two doses) when urine output was satisfactory.

Results

There was no donor mortality. The median blood loss of the donor operation was 500 ml (range 170–1600 ml). Only one donor, who had preexisting thalassemia, received one unit of homologous transfusion during the operation. The median duration of hospital stay was 10 days (range 5–38 days). A major complication occurred in six donors (7%) (all of whom were right-lobe donors). Donors 14, 23, and 76 developed cholestasis that eventually resolved. Donor 16 had biliary stricture at the confluence of the hepatic ducts. She recovered after a bilioenteric bypass at segment 3 of the hepatic duct. Donor 35 had a small bowel obstruction due to an adhesion band. She recovered after laparotomy and band division. Donor 49 had a bleeding duodeual ulcer which was controlled by heater probe applications. Thirteen donors had minor complications, including wound infection ($n = 10$), transient foot-drop ($n = 1$), a pressure sore ($n = 1$), and urinary tract infection ($n = 1$). The postoperative hemoglobin, INR, serum bilirubin, and aspartate aminotransferase of the right-lobe donors were compared with those of the left-lobe and left lateral segment donors (Figs. 5–8). Although the values of INR and serum

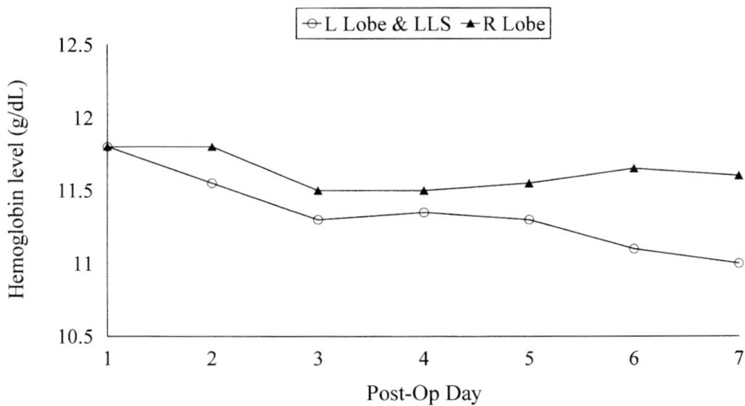

FIG. 5. Postoperative median hemoglobin concentrations in right-lobe and left-lobe donors

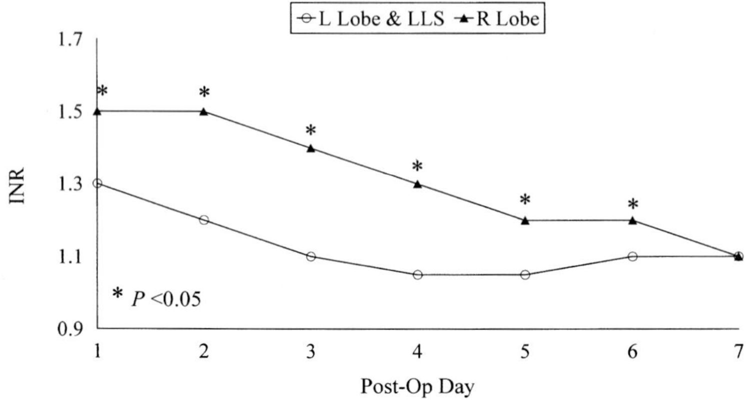

FIG. 6. Postoperative median international normalized ratio (*INR*) values of right-lobe and left-lobe donors

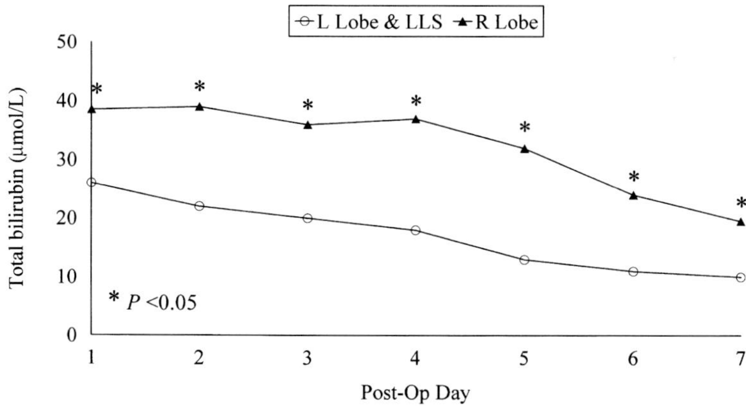

FIG. 7. Postoperative median serum bilirubin levels of right-lobe and left-lobe donors

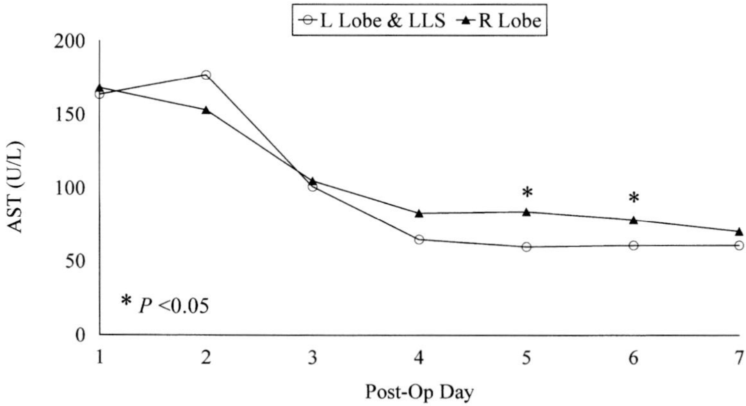

FIG. 8. Postoperative median values of aspartate aminotransferase in right-lobe and left-lobe donors

TABLE 3. Volume of liver graft and relationship between donors and recipients

	Graft type		
	Left lateral segment ($n = 16$)	Left lobe ($n = 6$)	Right lobe ($n = 66$)
Volume (g)	257.5 (165–515)	430 (343–623)	577.5 (390–1140)
% ESLM of recipient body weight	126.4 (32.9–203.2)	39 (31.5–72.4)	48.3 (32.8–88.7)
Body weight			
Donor > recipient	16	6	15
Donor = recipient	0	0	3
Donor < recipient	0	0	48

ESLM, estimated standard liver mass

bilirubin were generally worse in the right-lobe donors than in the left-lobe and left lateral segment donors, all right-lobe donors recovered uneventfully from the operation. The graft volumes and their ratios with the estimated standard liver masses of the recipients are given in Table 3. The right-lobe grafts provided more than 40% of the estimated liver mass in all except four recipients. The body weight of the right-lobe recipients was higher than that of the corresponding donors in 48 (73%) pairs.

The overall survival of the pediatric recipients was 75%. For the adults, when a left-lobe graft was used, the survival rate was 100% (3/3) for patients with fulminant hepatic failure, and 0% (0/2) for patients with cirrhosis. With the use of a right-lobe graft, the overall survival rate was 83% (55/66). Technical complications included hepatic vein stenosis ($n = 2$), portal vein stenosis ($n = 4$), hepatic artery stenosis ($n = 1$), biliary leakage ($n = 5$), and biliary stenosis ($n = 10$). The incidence of biliary stenosis was reduced from 30% in the first 30 operations to 3% in the last 36 operations as the result of a technique that preserves the blood supply to the right hepatic duct, accurately localizes the division of the right hepatic duct, and spaces the sutures appropriately. The causes of recipient mortality are shown in Table 4. There was no difference in the long-term survival of patients undergoing elective or emergency transplantation (Fig. 9).

Discussion

LDLT using a left-lobe graft or left lateral segment graft is an established procedure to overcome graft shortages, but it does not always benefit adult patients. The development of LDLT using a right-lobe graft is a promising

TABLE 4. Causes of mortality in recipients

Cause	Number
Pediatric patients	
Hepatic artery pseudoaneurysm[a]	1
Posttransplant lymphoproliferative disorder	1
Cytomegalovirus disease[a]	1
Hepatic vein stenosis	1
Adult patients	
Hepatic vein stenosis[a]	1
Intracerebral bleeding[a]	1
Fungal infection[a]	2
Primary graft nonfunction[a]	2
Thoracic empyema	1
Biliary leakage[a]	1
Biliary stenosis	1
Dissecting aortic aneurysm	1
Acute pancreatitis[a]	1
Legionella[a]	1
Thrombotic thrombocytopenic purpura[a]	1

[a] Hospital mortality

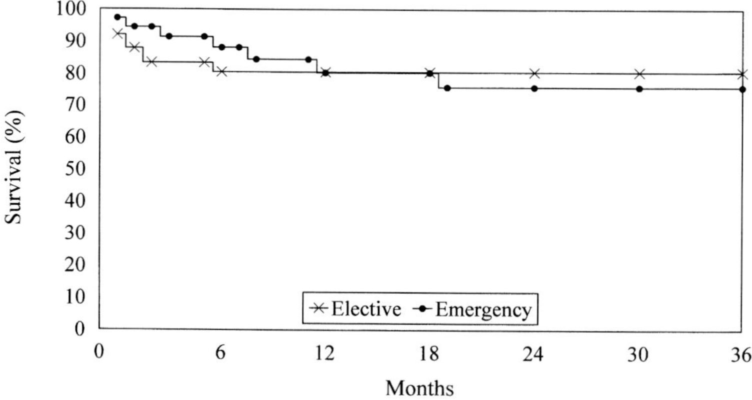

FIG. 9. Survival curves of patients receiving emergency and elective liver transplantation

solution but it has not been fully established because there are many unresolved technical issues. The use of a right-lobe graft in an LDLT was reported in 1994 by Yamaoka et al. [9]. It was performed in a pediatric patient, and the graft did not contain the middle hepatic vein. This chapter shows that with the inclusion of the middle hepatic vein, the authors have established a technique that can safely be applied to donors and is often of benefit to adult recipients. However, the inclusion of the middle hepatic vein in a right-lobe graft is controversial. The middle hepatic vein was routinely included in the graft in all our patients because it is the main drainage vein of segments V and VIII, and graft congestion was observed by us and in other reported series if the middle hepatic vein was not patent or not included in the graft [10, 11]. Routine inclusion of the middle hepatic vein in the graft will eliminate the necessity of excluding a donor with a small right hepatic vein and increase the applicability of the procedure [12]. As shown in this series, the inclusion of the middle hepatic vein in the graft did not induce liver failure in the donor. Cholestasis occurred in three donors, but overt clinical and biochemical manifestations of liver failure did not occur. If the segment IVb hepatic vein is retained with the donor, the liver function of the donor is not seriously impaired.

The other controversial issue is the technique of biliary reconstruction. In our early experience, the biliary complication rate was high. Similar experiences were reported from other centers [13, 14]. After repeated evaluations of each operation, we found that a lack of blood supply to the right hepatic duct, more than one hepatic duct orifice, and a tiny opening in the jejunum were the causes of biliary complications [7]. The blood supply to the right hepatic duct was derived from the right hepatic artery, arterial arcades within the bile duct wall, the left hepatic duct, and the common hepatic duct, hilar plate, and caudate lobe [15]. To preserve the blood supply after division of the right hepatic duct (by which the blood supply from the arterial arcade is interrupted), it is essential to avoid dissecting in the tissue plane between the right hepatic duct and the right hepatic artery. By modifying our technique, we could achieve low leakage and stenosis rates of bilioenteric anastomoses. However, the construction of the bilioenteric anastomosis could sometimes be difficult and entails an additional jejuno-jejunal anastomosis. Attempts have been made by other surgeons in recent years to construct duct-to-duct anastomosis. The long-term results of duct-to-duct anastomosis are not yet known, but this technique will conceivably replace bilioenteric anastomosis in the future.

As shown here, a right-lobe graft could provide sufficient volume for most adults even when the donor is smaller in body size than the recipient. It also provides a graft of excellent quality for patients with fulminant hepatic failure or acute exacerbation of chronic hepatitis B liver disease (see Tables 1 and 3).

In conclusion, the development of right lobe graft transplantation is a major advance in LDLT. With increasing experience and modifications in the technique, right-lobe LDLT, in a similar way to left-lobe or left lateral segment LDLT, will be a standard operation in the future.

References

1. Raia S, Nery JR, Mies S (1989) Liver transplantation from live donors. Lancet 2:497
2. Strong RW, Lynch SV, Ong TH, et al. (1990) Successful liver transplantation from a living donor to her son. N Engl J Med 322:1505–1507
3. Haberal M, Buyukpamukcu N, Telatar H, et al. (1992) Segmental living liver transplantation in children and adults. Transplant Proc 24:2687–2689
4. Hashikura Y, Makuuchi M, Kawasaki S, et al. (1994) Successful living-related partial liver transplantation to an adult patient. Lancet 343:1233–1234
5. Lo CM, Gertsch P, Fan ST (1995) Living unrelated liver transplantation between spouses for fulminant hepatic failure. Br J Surg 82:1037
6. Lo CM, Fan ST, Liu CL, et al. (1997) Adult-to-adult living donor liver transplantation using extended right-lobe graft. Ann Surg 226:261–270.
7. Fan ST, Lo CM, Liu CL (2000) Technical refinement in adult-to-adult living donor liver transplantation using right-lobe graft. Ann Surg 231:126–131
8. Fan ST, Lo CM, Liu CL, et al. (2000) Safety of donors in live-donor liver transplantation using right-lobe grafts. Arch Surg 135:336–340
9. Yamaoka Y, Washida M, Honda K, et al. (1994) Liver transplantation using a right lobe graft from a living related donor. Transplantation 57:1127–1130
10. Lee SG, Lee YJ, Park KM, et al. (1999) Anterior segment congestion of a right lobe graft in living donor liver transplantation and its strategy to prevent congestion (in Korean). J Korean Soc Transplant 13:213–218
11. Inomata Y, Uemoto S, Asonuma K, et al. (2000) Right lobe graft in living donor liver transplantation. Transplantation 69:258–264
12. Tanaka K, Kobayashi Y, Kiuchi T (2000) Current status of living donor liver transplantation in adults. Curr Opin Organ Transplant 5:74–79
13. Testa G, Malago M, Valentin-Gamazo C, et al. (2000) Biliary anastomosis in living related liver transplantation using the right liver lobe: techniques and complications. Liver Transplant 6:710–714.
14. Marcos A, Ham JM, Fisher RA, et al. (2000) Single-center analysis of the first 40 adult-to-adult living donor liver transplants using the right lobe. Liver Transplant 6:296–301
15. Vellar ID (1999) The blood supply of the biliary ductal system and its relevance to vasculobiliary injuries following cholecystectomy. Aust NZ J Surg 69:816–820

Middle Hepatic Vein Reconstruction in Living-Donor Liver Transplantation Using the Right Lobe

Sung Gyu Lee

The major limitation of adult–adult living donor liver transplantation (A–A LDLT) is graft size insufficiency. Frequently, a left lobe graft from a small donor cannot meet the metabolic demands of a larger recipient. To overcome this limitation many institutes have performed LDLT using a right lobe graft with varying results. However, right lobe graft with no middle hepatic vein (MHV) trunk might be complicated by severe congestion of the anterior segment. The need for MHV reconstruction when using a right lobe graft has not yet been clearly described in the literature. We have had experience with anterior segment congestion of a right liver lobe graft. Our first five right lobe grafts without an MHV trunk were transplanted to two patients with hepatitis B virus (HBV) cirrhosis, two with fulminant hepatic failure, and one with secondary biliary cirrhosis. The right liver grafts weighed 650–1000 g, which corresponded to 48%–83% of the recipient's standard liver volume. All accessory right hepatic veins (middle and inferior right hepatic veins) were anastomosed to the side of the recipient's vena cava. Immediately after portal reperfusion, extremely severe congestion and dusky discoloration of the anterior segment developed in two patients followed by prolonged massive ascites and severe liver dysfunction. One of the patients died of sepsis with progressive hepatic dysfunction 20 days after transplantation. Based on this experience, we realized that a right liver graft without an MHV trunk can cause severe congestion injury of the anterior segment (corresponding to segments 5 and 8 according to Couinaud's nomenclature) because the hepatic venous outflow of the anterior segment drains mostly into the MHV. This graft congestion can cause severe graft dysfunction and septic complications in extreme cases. An extended right lobe graft, with the additional venous drainage provided by the MHV (first introduced by S.T. Fan in Hong Kong) avoids this AS congestion problem and offers better graft function. However, LDLT using an extended

Department of General Surgery, Division of Hepatobiliary Surgery and Liver Transplantation, Asan Medical Center, Ulsan University, Seoul, Korea

right liver graft expands the extent of the donor operation and is an important ethical issue in LDLT. The congestion can be prevented as follows. Reconstruction of MHV drainage of the right lobe graft into the recipicient's venous system has been performed at our institution since 1998, and we named the procedure a modified right lobe graft. This graft not only provides a functioning liver mass comparable to an extended right lobe graft because it eliminates possible AS congestion, it lessens the risk to the donor because an extended right lobe graft may provoke congestion injury of some part of the medial segment of the remaining donor liver. For reconstruction of MHV drainage, all major (>5 mm in diameter) MHV tributaries were preserved during donor hepatectomy and reconstructed with the recipient's autogenous interposition vein grafts at the back table. These reconstructed autogenous interposition grafts were anastomosed to the recipient's middle or left hepatic veins and vena cava after right hepatic vein and portal vein anastomosis. There should be adequate functioning of the liver graft after 1 week because intrahepatic venous collateral of the congestive area can be expected to develop by day 7 after transplant. Additionally, the graft volume starts to regenerate immediately after transplantation. Our current results with the patency of the interposition vein graft suggest that better survival can be expected after A–A LDLT using a right lobe graft without an MHV trunk once MHV tributaries are reconstructed. From February 1997 to December 2000 a total of 195 A–A LDLTs were performed on 194 patients older than 20 years, with a less than 10% hospital death rate. The grafts used were a modified right lobe in 100, left lobe in 56, right lobe in 24, extended right lobe in 3, left lobe including caudate lobe in 3, dual left lobes in 8, and posterior segment in 1. It is not clear whether all right lobe grafts without an MHV trunk require MHV reconstruction. There have been many reports of successful results using a right liver graft without MHV reconstruction. During the same period in our study, 24 right liver grafts did not require reconstruction of MHV tributaries because they were small (<5 mm in diameter). Makuuchi (Tokyo University) suggested that reconstruction of MHV tributaries is indicated when (1) regurgitating blood flow cannot be seen between the peripheral tributaries of MHV and the right hepatic vein, and (2) the portal vein of the anterior segment reveals retrograde outflow for the hepatic arterial inflow, as seen by intraoperative ultrasonography. Reconstruction is also indicated if the volume of the discolored area in the anterior segment after portal reperfusion seems to exceed the safe limit of the remnant liver volume of the graft. However, it is impractical to reconstruct MHV tributaries in the recipient after anterior segment congestion develops. Reconstruction can be easily performed at bloodless bench surgery. Therefore, reconstruction of MHV tributaries from the anterior segment at the back table is recommended when the encountered MHV tributaries during donor hepatectomy are more than 5 mm in diameter.

Part 2
Viral Hepatitis and Liver Transplantation

Liver Transplantation for Hepatitis B and C

John J. Fung

Liver transplantation (LTx) is considered effective therapy for patients with end-stage liver disease. Unfortunately, the results of TLx for patients with chronic viral hepatitis has not been as promising as for other liver disorders. A high rate of hepatitis recurrence in the allograft leading to a high incidence of graft and patient loss have led many transplant centers to reassess the use of LTx in these groups. Current strategies to prevent hepatitis B and C viral (HBV, HBC) reinfection focus on identifying patients with a low risk of reinfection, specifically those with markers for a low level of or no viremia. Trials to convert "high risk" hepatitis patients to "low risk" status have been initiated with the aim to reduce the viral burden at the time of LTx. Antiviral agents or immunostimulatory therapy before or after LTx (or at both times) have been proposed as a means to minimize recurrence of hepatitis in the liver allograft. Although this approach has been effective for HBV infection (i.e., with the use of hepatitis B immune globulin and nucleoside analogs, specifically lamivudine), this approach has not been as effective for the prevention or treatment of HCV infection. Ongoing trials are assessing the use of antibodies to HCV during the early posttransplant period as well as the use of α-interferon and ribaviron. Despite the lack of overwhelming efficacy of these approaches for HCV, the impact of recurrent HCV following LTx is less significant, at least during the early posttransplant period. Although the focus has been on specific issues related to prevention or treatment of viral hepatitis in LTx patients, there are still a number of areas ripe for investigation. Controversies regarding the use of LTx for viral hepatitis have persisted despite an appreciation for the risks associated with the selection, prophylactic preparation, and treatment of candidates. The U.S. Department of Health and Human Services has now approved LTx for HBV infection, reflecting improvements made in the clinical arena. However, further advances are needed for HCV prophylaxis and treatment of recurrent hepatitis following LTx.

Thomas E. Starzl Transplantation Institute, University of Pittsburgh, PA, USA

Strategies for the Treatment of Hepatitis B and C After Liver Transplantation

ULF P. NEUMANN, DANIEL SEEHOFER, JAN M. LANGREHR, and PETER NEUHAUS

Summary. Hepatitis B- and C-related liver cirrhosis is the most common indication for liver transplantation. However, owing to the high frequency of recurrence of hepatitis, the morbidity and mortality of recipients with hepatitis B or C are high when compared with other indications such as alcoholic cirrhosis or Budd-Chiari syndrome. The spontaneous risk of viral recurrence in patients with hepatitis B has been effectively reduced by the use of hepatitis B immunoglobulin and lamivudine. In contrast to this, hepatitis C virus (HCV) recurrence is almost universal, although long-term survival is not low compared with other indications. Prophylactic or therapeutic regimens that alter the course of disease in HCV-positive patients do not exist, and with longer follow-up times the prevalence of HCV-related graft failure is likely to increase. New immunosuppressive regimens and antiviral treatments combining ribavarin and interferon α have to be investigated to reduce further the complications of HCV recurrence in the future.

Key words. Hepatitis B, Hepatitis C, Liver transplantation, Treatment

Introduction

Hepatitis B and C have emerged as the most common indications for orthotopic liver transplantation (OLT) [1–3]. However, the risk of death in recipients with hepatitis B or C is high when compared with other indications such as alcoholic cirrhosis or Budd-Chiari syndrome. This is a consequence of recurrent disease after OLT in patients with hepatitis B virus (HBV) or hepatitis C virus (HCV). The incidence, viral kinetics, and therapeutic approaches are

Chirurgische Klinik und Poliklinik, Charité, Campus Virchow-Klinikum, Humboldt Universität zu Berlin, Augustenburger Platz 1, 13353 Berlin, Germany

very different for these two indications. In OLT for HBV, a number of pro-phylactic and therapeutic protocols have been established in recent years, but there is a lack of effective agents in the treatment of HCV recurrence. Owing to initially poor results and expensive postoperative prophylaxis, hepatitis B, in particular, as an indication for liver transplantation is still a controversial issue.

Hepatitis B Virus

Hepatitis B Recurrence

Hepatitis B reinfection of the graft from extrahepatic sources [4] is a serious complication after OLT, and the disease then shows a faster progression than in nontransplant patients. Consequently, the development of HBV cirrhosis of the graft within a few months [5], and fulminant cases with the histology showing fibrosing cholestatic hepatitis, have been observed. Until the in-troduction of passive immunoprophylaxis, HBV recurrence was the most common cause of death in patients who had received a transplant as a result of chronic hepatitis B [6]. Therefore, hepatitis B was considered to be a con-traindication for liver transplantation in many centers. The risk of HBV recur-rence depends on factors such as the preoperative viral replication status of the recipient [1], co-infections with hepatitis D virus (HDV) or HCV, and the antiviral and immunosuppressive regimen after transplantation. Therapeutic options in cases of hepatitis B recurrence were limited, since interferon-α monotherapy, the standard treatment for chronic hepatitis B in a nontrans-plant setting, has no proven benefit after liver transplantation [7].

Passive Immunoprophylaxis

The outcome of liver transplantation in hepatitis B patients has been dra-matically improved by the introduction of passive immunoprophylaxis with hepatitis B immunoglobulin (HBIg) [8]. Long-term HBIg with a target anti-HBs titer of more than 100 U/l is now commonly accepted as effective means of preventing reinfection of the graft and improving survival rates. In con-trast, short-term HBIg application for 6 or 12 months was not effective in reducing hepatitis B recurrence rates [1]. However, even under indefinite HBIg administration, a significant percentage of patients develops reinfec-tion, ranging from 20% to 40% [1, 9] in different centers. In these patients, HBV recurrence is often based on the formation of virus mutants with an altered structure of the hepatitis B surface antigen (HBsAg) [10]. These muta-tions occur during prolonged HBIg administration, and might be partially prevented by high-dose passive immunoprophylaxis with antibody titers of more than 500 or 1000 U/l [11]. However, even under this high-dose HBIg administration, reinfection is not prevented in all patients. The major drawback of passive immunoprophylaxis are its high cost, which ranges from US$15000 to US$40000 per patient per treatment year, depending on the target antibody titer. A newer and less expensive approach is the active immunization of hepatitis B patients after a course of HBIg administration for 12 months or more. The first reports on this approach are promising [12], and the newer preS1 and preS2 vaccines, in particular [13], might improve the response rates of active immunization after transplantation.

Nucleoside Analogues

Apart from passive immunoprophylaxis, the options for the treatment of post-transplant hepatitis B were limited until recently. Within the past few years, new nucleoside analogues have expanded the therapeutic options for HBV after liver transplantation. Famciclovir and lamivudine, two oral nucleoside analogues, have strong antihepatitis B activity. The purine analogue famciclovir, which is the oral formulation of the active metabolite penciclovir, is activated by viral enzymes and leads to chain termination of the DNA. Antiviral effects have been found against herpes viruses and HBV. Since 1993, studies of famciclovir [14] in transplant and nontransplant patients have been carried out. The initial promising results, with a good suppression of viral replication, could not be confirmed in the long term because more than 80% of patients showed a relatively fast viral breakthrough during treatment. However, despite this disappointing virological result, in our own studies the survival of patients with hepatitis B recurrence after liver transplantation was improved by famciclovir treatment (Fig. 1). Unfortunately, prophylactic approaches with famciclovir in combination with HBIg did not achieve a reduction in recurrence rates (Fig. 2). In conclusion, famciclovir monotherapy or prophylaxis is not recommended for hepatitis B patients after liver transplantation, but studies are underway to discover whether famciclovir could have some role in antiviral combination treatment.

Very good results have been achieved with lamivudine treatment of hepatitis B reinfection. Lamivudine is a potent irreversible inhibitor of the reverse transcriptase (DNA polymerase). Studies in transplant recipients were started in 1996 and showed good supression of viral replication in more than 90% of our own patients ($n = 34$). Most of them became HBV DNA negative by hybridization assay, and liver enzymes decreased in parallel. Comparable results were obtained in a multicenter trial involving 52 patients. In this report by Perrillo et al. [15], 60% of patients became HBV DNA negative by hybridization assay and 6% seroconverted to HBsAg negativity. The antiviral activity of lamivudine is markedly higher than that of famciclovir [16], and lamivudine also shows suppression of viral replication in most, but not all, patients

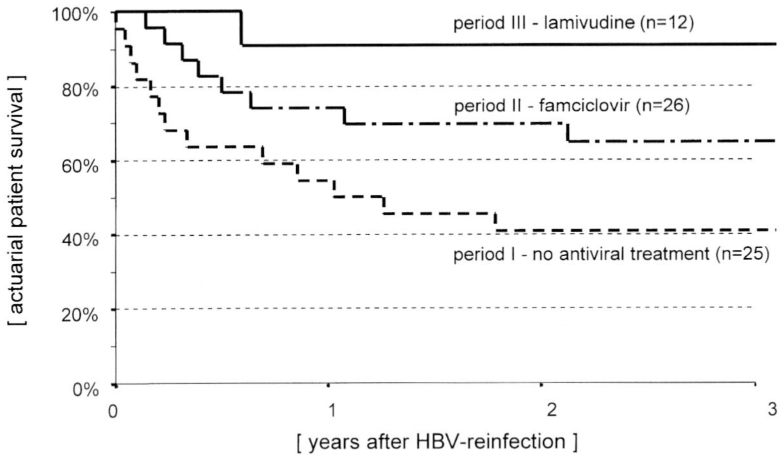

FIG. 1. Survival after hepatitis B reinfection in different antiviral periods

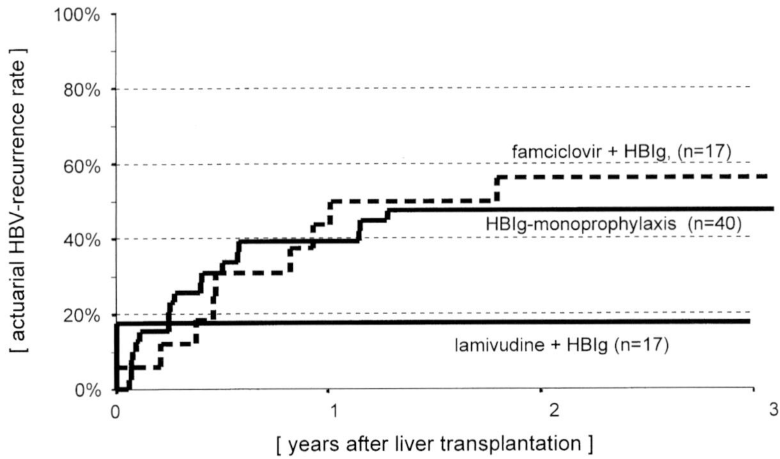

FIG. 2. Hepatitis B recurrence rates under hepatitis B immunoglobulin (*HBIg*) mono-prophylaxis compared with combination prophylaxis with HBIg plus famciclovir (*P* not significant) and with HBIg plus lamivudine (*P* < 0.05)

with famciclovir resistance. In addition, lamivudine has an excellent safety profile. Unfortunately, with lamivudine treatment, a significant percentage of patients (40%–60%) developed viral breakthrough within 2 years of treatment. At present, lamivudine is the treatment of choice for hepatitis B after transplantation. Whether it should be used as monotherapy or preferentially in combination with other antiviral agents (see below) has to be evaluated in future studies. The main problem is the development of resistance during prolonged treatment. If therapy is discontinued after the development of resistance, a reemergence of the wild-type virus with hepatitic flares has been reported [17]. Therefore, lamivudine treatment should not be discontinued [18], because with continuous treatment most breakthroughs result in only mild forms of hepatitis. In cases with an elevation in liver enzymes, rescue treatment with the addition of a second antiviral agent, e.g., interferon-α (IFN-α) or famciclovir, is successful in some, but not all, patients [19].

Recently, new nucleoside analogues with antihepatitis B activity have been developed, and these might open up new possibilities in cases of lamivudine resistance. At present, phase II/III studies with adefovir–dipivoxil [20] are ongoing in liver transplant patients with lamivudine resistance. The first in vitro results and results in a nontransplant setting show that adefovir is a very potent drug with activity against HBV even in cases of lamivudine resistance.

Viral Mutations

The major problems of antiviral treatment of hepatitis B infection after transplantation are the persistence of HBV and the development of resistance to the treatment. Viral persistence is mainly based on the incorporation of covalently closed circular DNA (CCC–DNA) in hepatic and extrahepatic reservoirs. Antiviral treatment is mostly ineffective against this viral replication state, and its elimination is only achievable by the immune system or by the death of the infected cells. The second problem is the relatively fast development of resistance by HBV in immunosuppressed patients. This is based on a high error rate in HBV DNA-polymerase owing to a lack of proofreading mechanisms. This favors single amino acid exchanges, which can lead to decreased sensitivity to antiviral agents. The incidence of lamivudine resistance in our own series was 55% after 2 years, and most resistance emerged during months 6–12 of treatment. The development of resistance is mostly based on mutations in HBV DNA-polymerase [21]. Most resistant genotypes have been identified as single amino acid exchanges at codon position 552, the so-called YMDD motif. They are sometimes associated with an additional mutation at codon 528. In general, these mutant viruses are thought to be replication defective [22]. Therefore, lamivudine-resistant reinfection is expected to have a milder clinical course, although clinical data are not available at present.

New problems will evolve in the future since antiviral agents are increasingly used in nontransplant settings, and potential recipients of liver grafts might already have shown lamivudine resistance prior to liver transplantation. Reinfection-free survival has been reported in such a case [23], but our own experience has shown early reinfection in 3 of 4 patients. Therefore, patients with preoperative lamivudine resistance represent problem cases after liver transplantation, and their optimal management has to be evaluated.

Combination Therapy

Multidrug regimens are already standard to prevent the development of resistance in therapy for human immunodeficiency virus infection. Synergistic combination regimens might also prevent resistance during antiviral treatment for HBV. A first step toward a combination of different agents is reinfection prophylaxis with HBIg plus lamivudine [24], which is used in many centers at present. With combination prophylaxis, recurrence rates were significantly reduced in our own series (see Fig. 2). Therefore, the current standard prophylaxis should consist of both agents, since with lamivudine [25] or HBIg monoprophylaxis, resistant viral strains evolve in a significant percentage of patients.

In cases of hepatitis B recurrence, combination therapy with lamivudine plus famciclovir or IFN-α can be recommended until the approval of new antiviral agents, such as adefovir. Whether combination therapy can significantly delay the development of resistance in comparison with sequential therapy with, e.g., famciclovir and lamivudine, must be confirmed in further studies.

Long-Term Results

Using these modern approaches of antiviral prophylaxis and treatment, excellent long-term results can also be achieved for hepatitis B patients. In our own series of 206 patients who were given transplants because of hepatitis B-related liver disease within the past 12 years, the overall 1-, 5-, and 10-year patient survival rates were 95%, 80%, and 75%, respectively.

Summary

At present, the recurrence of hepatitis B after liver transplantation is generally preventable with effective prophylaxis with HBIg and lamivudine. Thus, survival rates in hepatitis B patients are comparable to those of patients who have had transplants for other, nonviral indications. If reinfection occurs, early graft losses have become rare because of an increasing number of antiviral agents with antihepatitis B activity which can be used as monotherapy or in combination with other agents. If resistance against a single agent occurs, a change of therapy to another agent or a combination of different agents is often useful. However, new antiviral agents and other treatment strategies are on the horizon (Table 1), which raise new hopes for the future prophylaxis and treatment of hepatitis B after liver transplantation. Therefore hepatitis B patients, even with preoperative viral replication, should not be excluded from transplantation programs.

TABLE 1. Current and future therapeutic approaches for the treatment of chronic hepatitis B

Immunomodulators	Interferon-α
	Thymosin-α1
	Interleukin-2/interleukin-12
Nucleoside analogues	Ganciclovir
	Famciclovir
	Lamivudine
	Adefovir (nucleotide analogue)
	Lobucavir
Vaccination	PreS or S peptide vaccination
	Cytotoxic lymphocyte epitope vaccination
	DNA vaccination
Molecular therapy	Antisense oligonucleotides

Hepatitis C Virus

Hepatitis C has emerged as the most common indication for liver transplantation [3]. In contrast to HBV-related liver cirrhosis, the recurrence of HCV after OLT is almost universal [26]. The redistribution of the virus arises from extrahepatic sources [27]. Molecular analysis has shown that postoperative viral strains are identical to isolates detected before transplantation [28]. Following liver transplantation, the viral load increases more than 10-fold compared with pretransplant levels [29]. This is thought to reflect the suppression of the host effector immune response that usually controls HCV replication. This results in severe HCV-related graft hepatitis in nearly 50% of HCV-positive patients after OLT. Up to 15% of all HCV-positive patients develop cirrhosis in the course of the disease, but fewer than 5% will require retransplantation [30, 31]. An analysis of medium-term patient and graft survival figures showed no differences between OLT for HCV and OLT for other indications (Fig. 3). The main goal in the treatment of HCV-positive patients after OLT in the future is eradication of the viral infection, and the development of cirrhosis should also be prevented.

Outcome of HCV After OLT

Hepatitis C after OLT most commonly occurs during the first year posttransplant. The majority of liver transplant recipients show histological damage in liver biopsy specimens within this time [32]. Afterward, the progression of graft damage due to recurrent hepatitis is slow. Data on 8-year graft survival

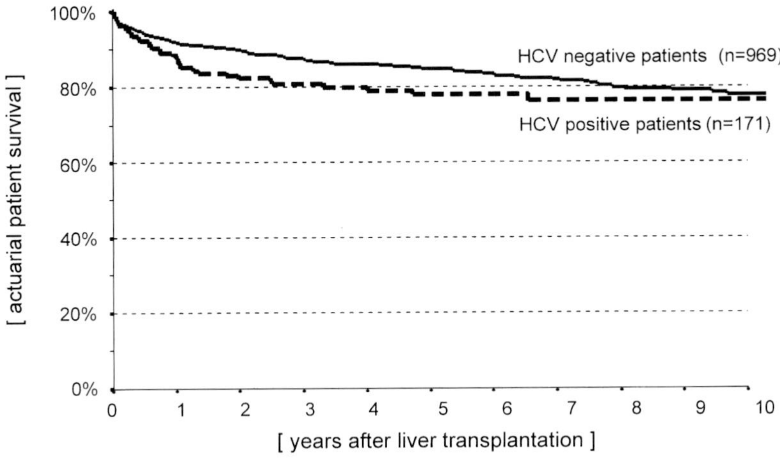

FIG. 3. Long-term survival was similar in HCV-positive patients when compared with other indications after OLT

rates do not show any differences between HCV-positive patients and those with other indications [33]. However, there is a lack of data analyzing longer follow-up periods, and these may be necessary to investigate the impact of recurrent HCV.

Several risk factors for the development and severity of graft hepatitis have been reported. A relationship between HCV viremia levels and genotype 1b has been suggested in the pathogenesis of severe recurrent hepatitis, but the matter remains controversial [34]. In most studies, the incidence of recurrent hepatitis C is similar in the 1b and non-1b groups, but genotype 1b is associated with more severe histological graft damage [35]. However, to date there is no evidence that graft survival is significantly lower in the genotype 1b group. Charlton et al. [36] reported that pretransplant HCV RNA titers $>10^6$ vEq/ml are associated with a lower rate of graft survival. These data could not be confirmed by others, who could not find an association between preoperative viremia levels and the outcome after OLT [34]. It had previously been shown that HCV envelope proteins correlate with viremia after OLT, but the clinical evidence of the impact of this correlation remains unclear [37].

Immunosuppression

Immunosuppression has to be divided into immunosuppressive induction protocols and rejection treatment. The incidence of acute and chronic rejection in HCV-positive patients has been reported to be higher than that for other indications [38]. The reasons for this are not yet clear, but in studies analyzing patients given transplants before 1990, in particular, acute rejection was often confounded with a recurrence of the disease. Current immunosuppressive induction protocols consist of calcineurin inhibitors (cyclosporin A [CsA], tacrolimus [Tac]), corticosteroids, mono- and polyclonal antibodies (interleukin-2 receptor antibodies), azathioprine, and mycophenolate mofetil (MMF).

The effect of CsA treatment on viremia in HCV-positive patients has been observed in nontransplantation patients. In a group of ten patients, no changes in viremia during the administration of 1.5–4 mg/kg CsA could be observed [39]. Although there are no data available for nontransplantation patients receiving Tac, in the posttransplant setting viremia in CsA- and Tac-treated patients receiving steroids are similar [40]. In addition, extensive studies could show no differences in the long-term outcome of Tac- and CsA-treated patients [30]. These data are confirmed by our own patient population, where long-term graft and patient survival figures were similar in patients receiving CsA and Tac. In contrast to CsA/Tac administration the use of steroids significantly increases the level of viremia in HCV-positive patients, and is related to histologic injury [41]. For this reason, we carried out a randomized trial of a steroid-free immunosuppressive induction protocol with MMF and Tac in 20 patients. The first results show that steroid-free induction therapy is safe and associated with a low incidence of rejections. Long-term data are awaited to show whether steroid-free immunosuppression induction protocols decrease the incidence and severity of recurrent graft hepatitis. MMF might be an alternative treatment option in HCV patients after OLT, because it has been shown to reverse acute rejection in HCV-positive recipients in the long term [42].

Furthermore, it has been suggested that MMF has some antiviral effects in vitro and in vivo [43]. This would mean that MMF should become the optimal immunosuppressant in HCV-positive liver transplant recipients. In contrast to these results, new data showed an increase in HCV viremia after OLT when MMF was added to the immunosuppressive treatment [44]. Recently, potent new immunosuppressants have been developed, and these might offer new possibilities for patients with HCV after OLT. Sirolimus, a macrocyclic lactone, has been investigated in large multicenter trials, and is reported to be more likely to inhibit viral infections. However, to date no data are available on the incidence of viral infections and sirolimus after OLT.

The standard first-line treatment of acute rejection after OLT still consists of steroid pulse therapy. Gane et al. [41] clearly demonstrated that steroid pulse therapy is associated with a 4–100-fold increase in HCV RNA levels and the subsequent development of acute hepatitis. RNA levels were significantly higher in patients with severe graft hepatitis in this study. Other researchers have reported similar findings. In a recent analysis of predictors for the outcome for patients after OLT for HCV, higher average doses of steroids and steroid treatment for acute rejection were associated with increases in graft loss and mortality [36]. OKT3 treatment for steroid-resistant acute rejection results in a shorter time interval to graft hepatitis and an increased rate of cirrhosis (26.3% vs. 6%) [45]. While the type of calcineurin inhibitor has no influence on the histologic recurrence of HCV, cumulative exposure to steroids and OKT3 is associated with an increased number of graft losses. A diagnosis of rejection in HCV-positive patients after OLT has to be made following rigorous criteria. Every effort should be made to enroll HCV-positive patients into studies that contribute to the optimization of pre- and post-transplant management.

Antiviral Therapy

Early studies used the biochemical response (i.e., the normalization of serum alanine aminotransferase [AST]) as the parameter of the efficacy of antiviral treatment. Currently, efficacy is also defined by the loss of HCV RNA in the serum. Two important new drugs have been introduced in the clinical setting after OLT. Ribavarin is a nucleoside analogue with a broad spectrum of action against DNA and RNA viruses. The most frequent side effect of ribavarin is hemolysis. In liver transplant recipients, the biochemical response achieved by ribavarin monotherapy appears to be greater than 50% [46]. In contrast, long-term investigations have shown no effect of ribavarin monotherapy on HCV viremia and the development of histological damage [46]. The biochemical and histological responses induced by IFN-α treatment of recurrent HCV after OLT are attributed to its direct antiviral effects. Despite initial virological response rates of 20%–50% in liver transplant recipients, most patients relapse after the withdrawal of therapy [47]. A similar lack of sustained response has been reported in renal transplant recipients, and probably reflects immunosuppression-enhanced viral replication. IFN-α has potent immunomodulatory functions and has been associated with an increased risk of rejection after OLT [48, 49]. Other severe side effects are leukopenia, nausea, and psychiatric disorders. Recent reports indicate that a combination of ribavirin and IFN-α is more effective than monotherapy in nontransplant patients. Up to 50% of patients eradicate viremia with ribavarin and IFN-α treatment [50]. In a large multicenter study of 122 liver transplant recipients, combination therapy was associated with an end-of-treatment biochemical and virological response in 35% of patients and a sustained virological response in 18% of patients 6 months after OLT. No differences were found between 6 months and 12 months of therapy. The recent introduction of new formulations of interferons (pegylated interferons) in the treatment of non-transplanted patients showed promising results. Monotherapy with pegylated interferons led to an virological response rate of more than 60%, and

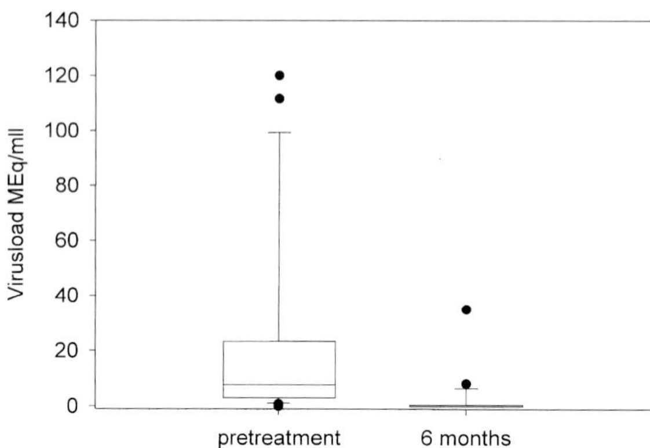

Fig. 4. Six months treatment with a combination of ribavarin and peginterferons led to a significant decrease in viremia in 25 HCV-positive patients with recurrent hepatitis after OLT

sustained response rates of 38% [51]. It can be expected that these results would be improved with a combination of ribavarin and pegylated interferons. For this reason, we started to treat patients with histologically proven graft hepatitis due to HCV with a combination of pegylated interferons and ribavarin. The results of our study are promising, with a virological response in more than 60% of patients and a biochemical response in more than 90% of patients after 30 weeks of treatment (Fig. 4). The side effects were leukopenia (60%), anemia (20%), psychiatric disorders (8%), and others (28%). However, there are few data concerning the sustained response owing to the limited follow-up period in this study. The optimal timing of antiviral therapy is not known, and is still a matter of discussion. A recent study suggests that the response to interferon/ribavirin is higher when therapy is started at the onset of acute hepatitis, rather than being delayed until 1 year posttransplant. The results of a study of antiviral therapy in hepatitis C patients have increased interest in attempting to eradicate the virus immediately prior to transplantation, as for patients with HBV. Theoretically, interferon therapy should be most effective when administered immediately after the transplantation when viremia is lowest [52]. In a recent study, patients received either IFN-α or no treatment after OLT. IFN-α decreased the incidence of graft hepatitis significantly 1 year after OLT (27% vs. 54%) [53]. However, the survival figures were similar in the two groups after 1 and 2 years.

Summary

Optimized immunosuppressive protocols are needed to improve the outcome in patients with HCV-related liver failure after OLT. Newer agents such as MMF and sirolimus have to be evaluated for their effects on viremia and the development of graft hepatitis posttransplantation. The treatment and prophylaxis of HCV recurrence will consist of interferons and ribavarin until new, more potent inhibitors of HCV replication become available. New treatment approaches with pegylated interferons may be a promising method for effectively reducing the complications of recurrent HCV after OLT. Another management option is passive immunoprophylaxis with immunoglobulins.

References

1. Samuel D, Muller R, Alexander G, et al. (1993) Liver transplantation in European patients with the hepatitis B surface antigen. N Engl J Med 329:1842–1847
2. Muller R, Samuel D, Fassati LR, et al. (1994) "EUROHEP" consensus report on the management of liver transplantation for hepatitis B virus infection. European Concerted Action on Viral Hepatitis. J Hepatol 21:1140–1143
3. Alter MJ (1997) Epidemiology of hepatitis C. Hepatology 26(3 Suppl 1):62–65
4. Omata M (1990) Significance of extrahepatic replication of hepatitis B virus. Hepatology 12:364–366
5. Demetris AJ, Todo S, Van Thiel DH, et al. (1990) Evolution of hepatitis B virus liver disease after hepatic replacement. Practical and theoretical considerations. Am J Pathol 137:667–676
6. Todo S, Demetris AJ, Van Thiel D, et al. (1991) Orthotopic liver transplantation for patients with hepatitis B virus-related liver disease. Hepatology 13:619–626
7. Rakela J, Wooten RS, Batts KP, et al. (1989) Failure of interferon to prevent recurrent hepatitis B infection in hepatic allograft. Mayo Clin Proc 64:429–432
8. Lauchart W, Muller R, Pichlmayr R (1987) Immunoprophylaxis of hepatitis B virus reinfection in recipients of human liver allografts. Transplant Proc 19:2387–2389
9. Devlin J, Smith HM, O'Grady JG, et al. (1994) Impact of immunoprophylaxis and patient selection on outcome of transplantation for HBsAg-positive liver recipients. J Hepatol 21:204–210
10. Protzer Knolle U, Naumann U, Bartenschlager R, et al. (1998) Hepatitis B virus with antigenically altered hepatitis B surface antigen is selected by high-dose hepatitis B immune globulin after liver transplantation. Hepatology 27:254–263
11. Sawyer RG, McGory RW, Gaffey MJ, et al. (1998) Improved clinical outcomes with liver transplantation for hepatitis B-induced chronic liver failure using passive immunization. Ann Surg 227:841–850
12. Sanchez Fueyo A, Rimola A, Grande L, et al. (2000) Hepatitis B immunoglobulin discontinuation followed by hepatitis B virus vaccination: a new strategy in the prophylaxis of hepatitis B virus recurrence after liver transplantation. Hepatology 31:496–501
13. McDermott AB, Cohen SB, Zuckerman JN, Madrigal JA (1998) Hepatitis B third-generation vaccines: improved response and conventional vaccine non-response—evidence for genetic basis in humans. J Viral Hepat 2:9–11
14. Main J, Brown JL, Howells C, et al. (1996) A double-blind, placebo-controlled study to assess the effect of famciclovir on virus replication in patients with chronic hepatitis B virus infection. J Viral Hepat 3(4):211–215
15. Perrillo R, Rakela J, Dienstag J, et al. (1999) Multicenter study of lamivudine therapy for hepatitis B after liver transplantation. Lamivudine Transplant Group. Hepatology 29:1581–1586
16. Rayes N, Seehofer D, Hopf U, et al. (2001) Comparison of lamivudine and famciclovir in the long-term treatment of hepatitis B infection following liver transplantation. Transplantation 71:96–101

17. Chayama K, Suzuki Y, Kobayashi M, et al. (1998) Emergence and takeover of YMDD motif mutant hepatitis B virus during long-term lamivudine therapy and re-takeover by wild type after cessation of therapy. Hepatology 27:1711–1716

18. Mutimer D, Pillay D, Shields P, et al. (2000) Outcome of lamivudine-resistant hepatitis B virus infection in the liver transplant recipient. Gut 46:107–113

19. Seehofer D, Rayes N, Berg T, et al. (2000) Additional interferon alpha for lamivudine-resistant hepatitis B infection after liver transplantation: a preliminary report. Transplantation 69:1739–1742

20. Perrillo R, Schiff E, Yoshida E, et al. (2000) Adefovir dipivoxil for the treatment of lamivudine-resistant hepatitis B mutants. Hepatology 32:129–134

21. Zoulim F, Trepo C (1998) Drug therapy for chronic hepatitis B: antiviral efficacy and influence of hepatitis B virus polymerase mutations on the outcome of therapy. J Hepatol 29:151–168

22. Melegari M, Scaglioni PP, Wands JR (1998) Hepatitis B virus mutants associated with 3TC and famciclovir administration are replication defective. Hepatology 27:628–633

23. Saab S, Kim M, Wright TL, et al. (2000) Successful orthotopic liver transplantation for lamivudine-associated YMDD mutant hepatitis B virus. Gastroenterology 119:481–486

24. Markowitz JS, Martin P, Conrad AJ, et al. (1998) Prophylaxis against hepatitis B recurrence following liver transplantation using combination lamivudine and hepatitis B immune globulin. Hepatology 28:585–589

25. Mutimer D, Pillay D, Dragon E, et al. (1999) High pre-treatment serum hepatitis B virus titre predicts failure of lamivudine prophylaxis and graft reinfection after liver transplantation. J Hepatol 30:715–721

26. Fukumoto T, Berg T, Ku Y, Bechstein WO, Hopf U, Neuhaus P (1997) Kinetics of hepatitis C viremia after orthotopic liver transplantation. Transplant Proc 29:511–513

27. Lerat H, Berby F, Trabaud MA, et al. (1996) Specific detection of hepatitis C virus minus strand RNA in hematopoietic cells. J Clin Invest 97:845–851

28. Arnold JC, Tox U, Goeser T, et al. (1997) Recurrent hepatitis C virus infection after liver transplantation—long-term follow-up with respect to the HCV genotypes/subtypes. Z Gastroenterol 35(4):255–261

29. Chazouilleres O, Kim M, Combs C, et al. (1994) Quantitation of hepatitis C virus RNA in liver transplant recipients. Gastroenterology 106:994–999

30. Gane EJ, Portmann BC, Naoumov NV, et al. (1996) Long-term outcome of hepatitis C infection after liver transplantation. N Engl J Med 334:815–820

31. Sheiner PA, Schluger LK, Emre S, et al. (1997) Retransplantation for recurrent hepatitis C. Liver Transplant Surg 3:130–136

32. Sheiner PA, Schwartz ME, Mor E, et al. (1995) Severe or multiple rejection episodes are associated with early recurrence of hepatitis C after orthotopic liver transplantation. Hepatology 21:30–34

33. Ghobrial RM, Farmer DG, Baquerizo A, et al. (1999) Orthotopic liver transplantation for hepatitis C: outcome, effect of immunosuppression, and causes of retransplantation during an 8-year single-center experience. Ann Surg 229:824–831

34. Berg T, Hopf U, Bechstein WO, et al. (1998) Pretransplant virological markers, hepatitis C virus genotype and viremia level are not helpful in predicting individual outcome after orthotopic liver transplantation. Transplantation 66:225–228

35. Gayowski T, Singh N, Marino IR, et al. (1997) Hepatitis C virus genotypes in liver transplant recipients: impact on posttransplant recurrence, infections, response to interferon-alpha therapy and outcome. Transplantation 64:422–426

36. Charlton M, Seaberg E, Wiesner R, et al. (1998) Predictors of patient and graft survival following liver transplantation for hepatitis C. Hepatology 28:823–830

37. Gane EJ, Maertens G, Ducatteeuw A, et al. (1999) Antibodies to hepatitis C virus envelope proteins correlate with hepatitis C viraemia after liver transplantation. Transplantation 67:78–84

38. Hoffmann RM, Gunther C, Diepolder HM, et al. (1995) Hepatitis C virus infection as a possible risk factor for ductopenic rejection (vanishing bile duct syndrome) after liver transplantation. Transplant Int 8:353–359

39. Kakumu S, Takayanagi M, Iwata K, Okumura A, Aiyama T, Ishikawa T, Nadai M, Yoshioka K (1997) Cyclosporine therapy affects aminotransferase activity but not hepatitis C virus RNA levels in chronic hepatitis C. J Gastroenterol Hepatol 12:62–66

40. Zervos XA, Weppler D, Fragulidis GP, et al. (1998) Comparison of tacrolimus with neoral as primary immunosuppression in hepatitis C patients after liver transplantation. Transplant Proc 30:1405–1406

41. Gane EJ, Naoumov NV, Qian KP, et al. (1996) A longitudinal analysis of hepatitis C virus replication following liver transplantation. Gastroenterology 110:167–177

42. Platz KP, Mueller AR, Willimski C, et al. (1998) Indications for mycophenolate mofetil therapy in hepatitis C-patients undergoing liver transplantation. Transplant Proc 30:1468–1469

43. Neyts J, Andrei G, De Clercq E (1998) The novel immunosuppressive agent mycophenolate mofetil markedly potentiates the antiherpesvirus activities of acyclovir, ganciclovir, and penciclovir in vitro and in vivo. Antimicrob Agents Chemother 42:216–222

44. Rostaing L, Izopet J, Sandres K, et al. (2000) Changes in hepatitis C virus RNA viremia concentrations in long-term renal transplant patients after introduction of mycophenolate mofetil. Transplantation 69:991–994

45. Rosen HR, Shackleton CR, Higa L, et al. (1997) Use of OKT3 is associated with early and severe recurrence of hepatitis C after liver transplantation. Am J Gastroenterol 92:1453–1457

46. Cattral MS, Hemming AW, Wanless IR, et al. (1999) Outcome of long-term ribavarin therapy for recurrent hepatitis C after liver transplantation. Transplantation 67:1277–1280

47. Gopal DV, Rabkin JM, Berk BS, et al. (2001) Treatment of progressive hepatitis C recurrence after liver transplantation with combination interferon plus ribavarin. Liver Transplant 3:181–190

48. Gadano AC, Mosnier JF, Durand F, et al. (1995) alpha-Interferon-induced rejection of a hepatitis C virus-infected liver allograft tolerated with a low dosage immunosuppressive regimen. Transplantation 59:1627–1629

49. Feray C, Samuel D, Gigou M, et al. (1995) An open trial of interferon alfa recombinant for hepatitis C after liver transplantation: antiviral effects and risk of rejection. Hepatology 22(4 Pt 1):1084–1089

50. Bizollon T, Palazzo U, Ducerf C, et al. (1997) Pilot study of the combination of interferon alfa and ribavarin as therapy of recurrent hepatitis C after liver transplantation. Hepatology 26:500–504

51. Zeuzem S, Feinmann SV, Rasenack J, et al. (2000) Peginterferon alfa-2a in patients with chronic hepatitis C. New Engl J 343:1666–1672

52. Christie JM, Healey CJ, Watson J, et al. (1997) Clinical outcome of hypogammaglobulinaemic patients following outbreak of acute hepatitis C: 2 year follow up. Clin Exp Immunol 110:4–8

53. Sheiner PA, Boros P, Klion FM, et al. (1998) The efficacy of prophylactic interferon alfa-2b in preventing recurrent hepatitis C after liver transplantation. Hepatology 28:831–838

Prophylaxis and Posttransplant Treatment of Viral Hepatitis in Living-Donor Liver Transplantation

Takafumi Ichida[1] and Yoshinobu Satoh[2]

Summary. Reinfection with hepatitis B virus (HBV) after liver transplantation (LT) causes both severe hepatitis and fibrosing cholestatic hepatitis (FSH) as early events, or liver cirrhosis within 5 years as a late event. Reinfection with hepatitis C virus (HCV) may not involve harmful events, but the majority of recipients develop chronic hepatitis and are at risk of hepatocellular carcinoma.

As prophylaxis for HBV, living-donor liver transplantation (LDLT) is designed to allow the administration of lamivudine for a period of about 2–3 months before LT. The administration of lamivudine should be continued after LT with hepatitis B immunoglobulin being maintained at over 500 IU/ml.

A prophylaxis for HCV has not yet been established. With cadaveric LT, we use both interferon and ribavirin for HCV, but it is not known for how long these drugs need to be administered before an adequate donor is available. Major complications are thrombocytopenia and hemolytic anemia. In our experience of the treatment of chronic hepatitis type C, the serum level of HCV-RNA decreases immediately after the administration of interferon-α and -β. Therefore, it is recommended that interferon-β be administered for 1–2 weeks before LDLT to obtain seronegative HCV-RNA.

Key words. Liver transplantation, Hepatitis B virus, Hepatitis C virus, Recurrence of hepatitis, Prophylaxis of hepatitis

---

[1] Department of Internal Medicine III, [2] Department of Surgery I, Niigata University School of Medicine, 754 Asahimachi Dori 1, Niigata 951-8510, Japan

Introduction

The first successful case of living-donor liver transplantation (LDLT) in adults was in 1993 [1]. Later, LDLT involving adults was conducted in a number of facilities, and the current total is close to 350 cases. LDLT provides two adults with liver function because of the regenerative capability of one liver; it is a lifesaving treatment.

One reason for the rapid increase in cases of LDLT between adults is simply that there are numerous adults with liver disease in Japan. Many have chronic liver diseases with morbidity due to viral hepatitis. The use of transplant care where patients have lapsed into progressive and irreversible hepatic failure, such as decompensated cirrhosis and hepatocellular carcinoma, has yet to be established. In programs of liver transplantation for viral hepatitis, the most important issue is preventing reinfection with the hepatitis B virus (HBV) or the hepatitis C virus (HCV), and how to manage posttransplant treatment. This chapter reviews the clinical significance of, and problems associated with, LDLT in relation to hepatitis viral-related recipients.

HBV-Positive Recipients

Cadaveric liver transplantation has been performed in HBV-infected recipients with fulminant hepatic failure as a result of acute infection, as well as those with cirrhosis or hepatocellular carcinoma due to chronic infection. One finding from these cases is that reinfection with HBV in the grafted liver frequently occurs, particularly in cases of chronic liver disease. Rapid and severe hepatitis, as well as fibrosing cholestatic hepatitis [2], are initiated, with fatal results [3, 4]. Even when the advance of cirrhosis is very recent, severe hepatitis is the result and the prognosis is extremely poor [5]. Adaptation of transplantation from cadaveric donors based on the concept of equitable organ sharing was ruled out owing to clinical findings of postoperative HBV reinfection and high early death rates for HBV-positive recipients. Nonetheless, around 1987, immunological defense mechanisms against HBV reinfection after transplantation were provided by the administration of hepatitis B immunoglobulin (HBIG) [6, 7]. Thus, transplant results for HBV-recipients improved, and the reverse-transcriptase inhibitor lamivudine appeared in 1995 [8]. As a result of this development, the long-term prognosis for HBV-positive cirrhosis recipients today [9] is extremely favorable [10].

From 1987 to 1995, transplantation results in the US gave an overall 8-year survival rate of 58%, although the 8-year survival rate for HBV-positive recipients of liver transplants was only 47%. Looking at recent European results [11], one can see that the overall results for liver transplants showed a 5-year survival rate of 67% after 1988; the 10-year survival rate was 61%. The results for all cases of HBV-positive cirrhosis compare favorably with these findings; the 5-year survival rate was 68% and the 10-year survival rate was 61%, showing the remarkable results which European centers have achieved.

It is clear that treatment with interferon, an antiviral agent used to combat reinfection with HBV, generally does not contribute to an improvement in that survival rate. Accordingly, the current consensus is that only HBIG and lamivudine can be used as treatment strategies to contribute to long-term survival after liver transplantation for HBV cirrhosis. Overall strategies can be separated into preventive and treatment strategies, as outlined below. Prophylaxis has been described as consisting of (a) continuous administration of lamivudine starting before transplantation and continuing thereafter, (b) continuous administration of HBIG after transplantation, and (c) lamivudine administration before and after transplantation with concurrent use of HBIG.

Prophylaxis with HBIG

The first treatment tool used was HBIG. This was reported in 1987 [12], and by 1993 Samuel et al. [13] reported having prevented almost 33% of postoperative reinfection using HBIG. However, in 1994 there was a European consensus recommending resistance to the use of this treatment owing to problems in preventing reinfection for HBV-DNA-positive cases [14]. Some problems with HBIG were also cited: (a) there is the risk of an allergic reaction as a result of intravenous injection; (b) the pharmokinetics are complicated as well as expensive; (c) there is the possibility of unknown viral infections because the drug is produced from human blood. Furthermore, the fact that the HBIG currently in use is not heat-treated is common knowledge.

However, reinfection can be prevented if an appropriate antibody titer can be maintained. There are many cases where survival has been prolonged without reduced quality of life (QOL) through the avoidance of HBV reinfection with continuous administration, albeit at a high price. Recent reports (Table 1) show that the objective of prolonging survival can be achieved if an appropriate hepatitis B surface antigen (HBsAg) titer is maintained [15, 16].

Prophylaxis with Lamivudine

The effects of lamivudine in HBV were reported in 1995 [8], and long-term survival was achieved through the use of lamivudine, independently and in combination with HBIG, to prevent reinfection. This treatment began immediately for liver transplant recipients [9]. At the same time, lamivudine had a clinical application as an antiviral treatment that proved effective even during reinfection. Lamivudine was administered independently before transplantation to prevent reinfection. In about 70%–75% of cases of postoperative inde-

TABLE 1. Recent reports of prophylaxis of hepatitis B virus (HBV) with hepatitis B immunoglobulin (HBIG) monotherapy

Reference	Prophylaxis	Period	Titer of anti-HBsAg
McGory et al. [15]	25/25	2–55 months	>500 (0–7 day) >250 (8–90 day) >100
Tchervenkov et al. [16]	12/13	9–56 months	>1000

HBsAg, hepatitis B surface antigen

TABLE 2. HBV prophylaxis with lamivudine monotherapy for liver transplantation (LT)

Reference	Prophylaxis HBV(−)	Before LT dose (period)	After LT follow-up period	LT
Grellier et al. [17]	9/12 (75%)	100 mg (4 months)	18–90 weeks	Cadaver
Lo et al. [18]	9/12 (75%)	100 mg (4 months)	2–14 months	Cadaver
Perrillo et al. [19]	24/34 (71%)	100 mg (80 days)	52 weeks	Cadaver
Niigata	1/1 (100%)	100 mg (2 months)	52 weeks	Living

pendent administration, a decrease in the amount of HBV-DNA was seen. The dose was 100 mg given from about 80 to 120 days before transplantation, and continued after transplantation (Table 2). The prevention of reinfection by independent administration was successful in three-quarters of the cases [17–19]. However, one problem was that a mutant appeared in the YMDD motif, although this factor was determined not to be a lethal pathology. Nonetheless, future investigation in relation to this variation is necessary.

Prophylaxis with Lamivudine and HBIG

Markowitz et al. [20] administered 150 mg lamivudine before transplant, and the same amount in combination with HBIG after transplant. With the longest period of observation being 525 days, they reported that none of the 14 cases had anti-HBsAg and there were no HBV-DNA-positive cases [20]. Gugenheim et al. [21] used the combined administration of 100 mg lamivudine and 10 000 IU HBIG after transplantation in four cases, and although HBV infection was present after 2 months, it was not found to be present later. Naomov et al. [22] switched from the expensive HBIG to lamivudine only over the 6 months period after transplantation, and the clinical usefulness of this approach was noted.

In all recent reports, long-term follow-up had not been possible, and this led to difficulties in discussing the long-term prognosis. It is clear that HBV reinfection after transplantation in a form such as severe hepatitis is suppressed.

Accordingly, the prophylaxis strategy can be considered to lead to a good long-term prognosis. To date, the most effective prophylaxis treatment strategy with respect to anti-HBe and HBV-DNA-positive cases is priming with lamivudine before transplant, continuous administration postoperatively, and postoperative HBIG where recommended.

Posttransplant Treatment with Lamivudine

After considering the long-term prognosis, it is important to decide on an effective antiviral treatment strategy for cases of HBV infection occurring after liver transplantation. Lamivudine is currently administered as an antiviral agent after liver transplantation in the hope that a similar prognosis for long-term survival as that for regular chronic hepatitis will be achieved.

When Perillo et al. [23] administered lamivudine to HBV-positive recipients after transplantation, they eliminated anti-HBs in 8% of cases, anti-HBe in 31% of cases, and HBV-DNA in 60% of cases. They also found that laboratory measures of liver function improved. While this research had only a short-term follow-up, it is a critical study in terms of expectations for long-term prognoses. The finding that reinfection did not occur after liver transplantation is important in the clinical sense as well as for the QOL of recipients.

HCV-Positive Recipients

HCV Reinfection

HCV reinfection occurs at high rates after liver transplantation in HCV-positive recipients. This infection also occurs very soon after transplantation, and in many cases HCV-RNA can be detected in blood 2–4 weeks posttransplant. However, not all HCV-positive recipients will become HCV-RNA-positive after transplantation, and approximately 5% avoid reinfection. Although the reports show some differences, hepatitis is found histologically in 14%–72% of those reinfected [24, 25]. The author investigated 20 cases of liver transplantation to Japanese recipients from cadaveric donors in other countries. A later search for HCV-positive recipients living in Japan showed that all of these 20 cases had HCV-positive chronic hepatitis after liver transplantation [26, 27].

HCV reinfection and hepatitis occur at high rates in HCV-positive recipients, and this may have some effect on liver transplantation results. After reviewing all the research published to date, no significant difference was found between the 5-year survival rate for HCV-positive recipients after transplantation and that for other non-HCV-positive recipients [28–32] (Table 3).

TABLE 3. Hepatitis C virus (HCV)-infected recipients, noninfected recipients, and variation in survival rates

Researcher and year	Infection (no. of patients)	1-year survival (%)	5-year survival (%)	*P* value
Ferray 1994 [28]	HCV (79)	95	80	
	Non-HCV (106)	98	89	NS
Gane 1996 [29]	HCV (149)	79	70	
	Non-HCV (623)	75	69	NS
Boker 1997 [30]	HCV (61)		62	
	Non-HCV (474)		57	NS
Casavilla 1998 [31]	HCV (183)	80	75	
	Non-HCV (556)	78	70	NS
Ghobrial 1999 [32]	HCV (183)	86	76	
	Non-HCV (556)	81	71	NS

TABLE 4. Appearance of infection after liver transplantation, initiation of hepatitis, and severity-related factors

HCV viremia high titer before liver transplant
HCV quasispecies
HLA-related factors
   HLA B1, DRB1*04, DRB1 mismatch
   HLA DRB3
Macrovascular steatosis
Donor TNF-α polymorphism
IgM anti-HCV core antibody
Genotype I
HLA class II-restricted CD4 (+) T lymphocytes

HLA, human leukocyte antigen; TNF-α, tumor necrosis factor α

Nonetheless, there are cases where fibrosing cholestatic hepatitis is observed with HBV and cases where severe hepatitis is produced, as well as some cases involving a short-term transition to cirrhosis. The causes are unclear, and a number of reports suggest a relationship between many of the factors (Table 4). The factors involved in future HCV reinfection and the increasing severity of the hepatitis have not yet been clarified, and currently it is not possible to make definite conclusions.

TABLE 5. Treatment strategies with respect to recurrence of HCV after liver transplantation and results

	Dose	No.	BR (%)	PCR(−)	Hx;improv. (%)	Rejection (%)
Wright (H)	IFN 3MU × 3/W (6 months)	11	9	0	0	0
Wright (T)	IFN 3MU × 3/W (4 months)	18	28	0	0	4
Ferray	IFN 3MU × 3/W (6 months)	14	23	0	14	35
Cattral	Ribavirin (6 months)	9	44	0	22	0
Gane	Ribavirin (6 months)	7	57	0	57	0
Bizollon	IFN 3MU × 3/W + ribavirin (6 months)	21	100	48%	100	0

PCR, polymerase chain reaction; IFN, interferon

TABLE 6. Prophylaxis of HCV reinfection by interferon (IFN) and ribavirin (IFN 3 weeks after liver transplant, ribavirin 10 mg/kg/day started with meals)

	Dose	Graft	Hepatitis (%)	Clearance of HV (%)
Mazzaferro	IFN 3MU × 3/W + ribavirin	21	19	42
	IFN 3MU × 3/W	10	100	20
	No treatment	17	70.5	0

Prophylaxis for HCV Reinfection

HCV reinfection occurs at high rates after liver transplantation in HCV-positive recipients, although it does not seem to affect survival rates. However, a transition to severe hepatitis and cirrhosis in a short period of time has been noted recently, and thus HCV prophylaxis and treatment after liver transplantation have been considered. Interferon-α, which serves as a treatment tool against reinfection in HCV-positive recipients, was first used, but the results were poor [33, 34] and there was suspicion as to whether rejection was being elicited [35]. However, in recent years ribavirin has been administered in combination with interferon. When the administration of ribavarin alone [36, 37] was compared with the combined administration, it was found that the combination regimen led to dramatic improvements in treatment results [38]. Thus, it is believed to be a promising addition to the antiviral treatment strategy after transplantation (Table 5). The ideal situation would be to find no reinfection after liver transplantation, and the main thrust of current research is the administration of antiviral agents before transplantation. However, thrombocytopenia and a number of other complications make the planned administration of such agents before liver transplantation from a cadaveric donor difficult. The administration of interferon and ribavirin immediately after liver transplantation is successful in the prevention of reinfection. Mazzafero et al. [39] reported limiting HCV reinfection immediately after liver transplantation to 42% using combination therapy; however, the survival rate after 2 years was the same as that of the untreated group (Table 6).

References

1. Ichida T, Matsunami H, Kawasaki S, et al. (1995) Living related donor liver transplantation from adult to adult for primary biliary cirrhosis. Ann Intern Med 122:275–276
2. Davis SE, Portmann BC, O'Grady JG, et al. (1991) Hepatic histological findings after transplantation for chronic hepatitis B virus infection, including a unique pattern of fibrosing cholestatic hepatitis. Hepatology 13:150–157
3. Todo S, Demetris AJ, Van Theil DH, et al. (1991) Orthotopic liver transplantation for patients with hepatitis B virus-related liver disease. Hepatology 13:619–626
4. Belle SH, Beringer KC, Detre KM (1997) Recent findings concerning liver transplantation in the United States. In: Cecka JM, Terasaki PI (eds) Clinical transplants. UCLA Tissue Typing Laboratory, LA, pp 15–29
5. Chazouilleres O, Mamish D, Kim M, et al. (1994) "Occult" hepatitis B virus as source of infection in liver transplant recipients. Lancet 343:142–146
6. Lauchart W, Muller R, Pichlmayr R (1987) Immunoprophylaxis of hepatitis B virus reinfection in recipients of human liver allografts. Transplant Proc 19:2387–2388
7. Samuel D, Bismuth A, Mathieu D, et al. (1991) Passive immunoprophylaxis after liver transplantation in HBsAg-positive patients. Lancet 337:813–816
8. Dienstag JL, Perrillo RP, Schiff EF, et al. (1995) A preliminary trial of lamivudine for chronic hepatitis B infection. N Engl J Med 333:1657–1661
9. De Man RA, Niester HGM, Fevery J, et al. (1995) Evaluation of limiting dilution PCR of HBV-DNA decrease in a double-blind randomized six-month trial of lamivudine for chronic hepatitis B: Implications for application in liver transplant recipients. American Association for the Study of Liver Disease Single-Topic Symposium: Liver Transplantation for Chronic Viral Hepatitis, Hepatology, p 10 (abstract)
10. Ichida T, Satoh Y, Kashida H (2000) Long-term follow-up study of HBV-positive recipients after liver transplantation. Kan Tan Sui 41:131–138
11. European Liver Transplant Association (2000) In: European Liver Transplant Registry. Data Analysis Booklet May 1968 to December 1999
12. Lauchart W, Muller R, Pichlmayr R (1987) Long-term immunoprophylaxis of hepatitis B virus reinfection in recipients of human liver allograft. Transplant Proc 19:4051–4052
13. Samuel D, Muller R, Alexander G, et al. (1993) Liver transplantation in European patients with the hepatitis B surface antigen. N Engl J Med 329:1842–1847
14. Muller R, Samuel D, Fassati LR, et al. (1994) "EUROHEP" consensus report on the management of liver transplantation for hepatitis B virus infection. J Hepatol 21:1140–1143

15. McGory RW, Ishitani MB, Oliveira WM, et al. (1996) Improved outcome of orthotopic liver transplantation for chronic hepatitis B cirrhosis with aggressive passive immunization. Transplantation 61:1358–1364
16. Tchervenkov JI, Tector AJ, Barkun JS, et al. (1997) Recurrence-free long-term survival after liver transplantation for hepatitis B using interferon-alpha pretransplant and hepatitis B immune globulin posttransplant. Ann Surg 226:356–369
17. Grellier L, Mutimer D, Ahmed M, et al. (1996) Lamivudine prophylaxis against reinfection in liver transplantation for hepatitis B cirrhosis. Lancet 348:1212–1215
18. Lo CM, Fan ST, Lai CL, et al. (1999) Lamivudine prophylaxis in liver transplantation for hepatitis B in Asia. Transplant Proc 31:535–536
19. Perrillo RP, Schiff ER, Dienstag JL, et al. (1999) Lamivudine for prevention of recurrent hepatitis B after liver transplantation: final results of a U.S./Canadian multicenter trial. Hepatology 30:222A
20. Markowitz JS, Martin P, Conrad AJ, et al. (1999) Prophylaxis against hepatitis B recurrence following liver transplantation using combination lamivudine and hepatitis B immune globulin. Hepatology 28:585–589
21. Gugenheim J, Baldini E, Ouzan D, et al. (1999) Good results of lamivudine in hepatitis B surface antigen-positive patients with active viral replication before liver transplantation. Transplant Proc 31:554–555
22. Naomov NV, Lopes R, Crepalid G, et al. (1999) Randomized trial of lamivudine versus hepatitis B immunoglobulin for prophylaxis of HBV recurrence after liver transplantation. J Hepatol 50(S):51
23. Perrillo R, Rakela J, Dienstag J, et al. (1999) Multicenter study of lamivudine therapy for hepatitis B after liver transplantation. Hepatology 29:1581–1586
24. Bizollon T, Mutimer D, Ducerf C, et al. (1999) Hepatitis C virus recurrence after liver transplantation. Gut 44:575–578
25. Teixeira R, Pastacaldi S, Papatheodoridis GV, et al. (2000) Recurrent hepatitis C after liver transplantation. J Med Virol 61:443–454
26. Ichida T (1996) Clinical aspects of HCV after organ transplantation. Annual Report of Intractable Hepatic Diseases by Ministry of Health and Welfare 1995, pp 112–115
27. Ichida T (1997) Clinical problems of cadaveric liver transplantation for Japanese recipients. Acta Hepatol Jpn 38:129–133
28. Ferray C, Gigou M, Samuel D, et al. (1994) The course of hepatitis C virus infection after liver transplantation. Hepatology 20:1137–1143
29. Gane EJ, Portmann BC, Naoumov NV, et al. (1996) Long-term outcome of hepatitis C infection after liver transplantation. N Engl J Med 334:815–820
30. Boker KHW, Dalley G, Bahr MJ, et al. (1997) Long-term outcome of hepatitis C virus infection after liver transplantation. Hepatology 25:203–210
31. Casavilla FA, Rakela J, Kapur S, et al. (1998) Clinical outcome of patients infected with hepatitis C virus infection on survive after primary liver transplantation under tacrolimus. Liver Transplant Surg 4:448–454
32. Ghobrial RM, Farmer DG, Baquerizo A, et al. (1999) Orthotopic liver transplantation for hepatitis C. Outcome, effect of immunosuppressant, and causes of retransplantation during an 8-year single-center experience. Ann Surg 6:824–833
33. Wright HI, Gavaler JS, Van Thiel DH, et al. (1992) Preliminary experience with alpha-2b-interferon therapy of viral hepatitis in liver allograft recipients. Transplantation 53:121–124
34. Wright TL, Combs C, Kim M, et al. (1994) Interferon-alpha therapy for hepatitis C virus infection after liver transplantation. Hepatology 20:773–779

35. Feray C, Samuel D, Gigou M, et al. (1995) An open trial of IFN-alpha recombinant for hepatitis C after liver transplantation: antiviral effects and risk of rejection. Hepatology 22:1084–1089
36. Cattral MS, Krajden M, Wanless IR, et al. (1996) A pilot study of ribavirin therapy for recurrent hepatitis C virus infection after liver transplantation. Transplant 61:1483–1488
37. Gane EJ, Tibbs CJ, Ramage JK, et al. (1995) Ribavirin therapy for hepatitis C infection following liver transplantation. Transplant Int 8:61–64
38. Bizollon T, Palazzo U, Ducerf C, et al. (1997) Pilot study of the combination of alpha-interferon and ribavirin as therapy of recurrent hepatitis C after liver transplantation. Hepatology 26:500–504
39. Mazzafero V, Regalia E, Pulvirenti A, et al. (1997) Prophylaxis against HCV recurrence after liver transplantation. Effect of interferon and ribavirin combination. Transplant Proc 29:519–521

Part 3
Current Status and Future Prospects in Small Bowel Transplantation

Intestinal Transplantation

Alan N. Langnas

Summary. Intestinal transplantation has developed into an acceptable form of therapy for patients with life-threatening complications of intestinal failure. Intestinal failure is most commonly the result of loss of the gastrointestinal tract, which results in the short-bowel syndrome. The most common reason to consider patients for intestinal transplantation is when they have developed total parenteral nutrition-related liver disease. The type of transplant that the patient will receive is often dictated by the degree of underlying liver disease. Other indications for isolated intestinal transplantation include recurrent sepsis and loss of venous access. The surgical techniques for intestinal transplantation have been modified over the years. Patients are matched with donors based on blood type and size. Following transplantation, immune suppression is based on tacrolimus. Improvements in rejection episodes have been seen with the addition of interleukin-2-receptor blocking agents. Bowel biopsies are critical to making a diagnosis of rejection. Serious complications such as cytomegalovirus infections and lymphoproliferative disease are being managed with greater success. Chronic rejection remains a difficult long-term problem. The intestinal allograft can effectively provide nutritional autonomy to patients. As the results of intestinal transplantation continue to improve, more patients will be offered this form of therapy for treatment of their intestinal failure.

Key words. Small bowel, Transplantation, Intestinal, Failure, Isolated

Small bowel and small bowel/liver transplantation have evolved from an experimental therapy to an accepted form of treatment for patients with

Section of Transplantation, Department of Surgery, University of Nebraska Medical Center, 983285 Nebraska Medical Center, Omaha, NE 68198-3285, USA

intestinal failure with associated life-threatening complications, such as total parenteral nutrition (TPN)-associated liver disease. The Healthcare Financing Administration (HCFA) in the USA (Medicare) recently listed intestinal transplantation an approved form of therapy for intestinal failure [1]. Factors that have contributed to improved patient and allograft survival include new immunosuppressive agents, better patient selection, and refinements in the surgical procedure.

Parenteral nutrition (PN), developed in the early 1970s, became a life-saving therapy for patients with intestinal failure, particularly those with short-bowel syndrome. During the past 30 years PN, and particular home PN, has become a reasonably safe and effective way to provide nutritional support to patients with an absent or nonfunctioning gut. While most patients receiving long-term PN do well, there remains a subgroup of patients who will develop life-threatening complications, which include liver dysfunction, catheter-related sepsis, and central venous thrombosis. The North American Registry of patients on home PN demonstrates that the 1- and 4-year mortality rates for patients with short-bowel syndrome are 94% and 80%, respectively [2]. The survival rate for patients with functional disorders of the small bowel is even lower. It has also been estimated that 40%–60% of infants who become permanently dependent on PN will develop PN-related liver disease [3].

The current indications for intestinal transplantation include life-threatening complications of PN [4]. The most common reason for considering intestinal transplantation is the development of PN-induced liver disease. For patients with irreversible forms of PN-induced liver disease, combined liver/small bowel transplantation is indicated. For those patients in whom the liver disease is believed to be reversible, isolated small-bowel transplantation should be considered. The other two most common indications for isolated intestinal transplantation are recurrent episodes of sepsis and loss of venous access. The degree of sepsis is often difficult to quantify. A good guideline is those patients who have had multiple episodes of sepsis requiring not only admission to the hospital, but monitoring in an intensive care unit (ICU) and possibly the use of vasopressors. When patients are considered for transplantation due to loss of venous access, this typically suggests an inability to place central catheters in the internal jugular or subclavian veins. Also, the need for the placement of catheters in (extemporaneous) sites such as the femoral vein and the inferior vena cava, and transhepatically, are indications for isolated intestinal transplantation. Other less frequent indications for intestinal transplantation include locally aggressive tumors (desmoid) and a non-reconstructable gastrointestinal (GI) tract.

The evaluation of a patient with intestinal failure for intestinal transplantation includes the participation of a multidisciplinary group of healthcare professionals, including transplant surgeons, gastroenterologists, social workers, nurse specialists, and dietitians. Part of the evaluation process is an assessment of the patient's current feeding program. A thorough assessment of the GI tract is required, often involving both contrast studies and endoscopies. If liver disease is present, liver biopsies are useful in determining the degree and reversibility of the disease.

Once the evaluation is complete, and it is determined that a patient requires intestinal transplantation, he or she is placed on our transplant waiting list. Potential organ donors are matched with patients on our intestinal transplant waiting list based on blood type, size, and medical urgency according to United Network for Organ Sharing guidelines. The donor is typically 50% –70% of the size of the recipient, particularly for recipients who have short-bowel syndrome. If possible, recipients are matched with ABO-identical donors, although exceptions have been reported [5]. The cytomegalovirus (CMV) status of the donor is important. While a donor who is CMV positive is not a contraindication to the use of the organs, it is important in selecting the appropriate recipient. Typically, placing a CMV-positive organ into a CMV-negative recipient is reserved for those patients who are most desperately in need of liver/small bowel transplantation. At the University of Nebraska Medical Center, all organ donors are treated with both OKT3 and antithymocyte globulin in an attempt to immunomodulate the potential allograft. Currently we do not use osmotic agents to flush the intestinal contents or any specific intestinal decontamination regimen.

The surgical procedures for both isolated small bowel transplantation and combined liver/small bowel transplantation have been well described [6, 7]. Typically, for the isolated small-bowel donor, the abdomen is entered and the dissection is initiated by taking down the falciform ligament and the left triangular ligament, followed by mobilization of the right colon. An extensive Kocher maneuver will then help to expose the aorta and vena cava. When removing only the isolated small bowel, the dissection is directed toward the liver hilum. The bile duct is ligated and the gall bladder excised and flushed. The hepatic arterial anatomy is then identified. Once the dissection is complete, the pylorus is transected with a GI stapling device, as is the terminal ileum. The stomach and right colon are mobilized to the left. At this point, the donor is heparinized and the organs are flushed with University of Wisconsin solution through the aortic cannula. The amount of University of Wisconsin solution depends on the size of the organs. Slush may then be distributed in the abdominal cavity. Following this, the liver and small bowel are removed en bloc. The organs are then separated on a second operating table. The arterial supply is separated at the aorta so that the celiac access remains with the liver and the superior mesenteric artery with the small-bowel graft. In the event that there was a replaced right hepatic artery at the superior mesenteric artery, the superior mesenteric artery will be left with the liver graft. The portal vein is transected at the level of the duodenum.

The back table preparation of the isolated small-bowel graft involves removing the pancreas and duodenum from the portal vein and superior mesenteric arteries. With the completion of this dissection, the small-bowel graft remains with the staple line at the jejunum and terminal ileum. There should be a reasonable length of superior mesenteric artery and portal vein. An extension iliac artery graft may be required in some cases. (Fig. 1)

The procurement for a liver/small-bowel graft is similar to that for isolated small-bowel transplantation. The retroperitoneal exposure is identical. The supraceliac aorta does not need to be isolated for the liver/small-bowel procurement, as the whole thoracic aorta will be harvested en bloc with the abdominal segment comprising the celiac trunk and the superior mesenteric artery. There is no perihepatic dissection except for flushing the gall bladder. When removing the donor specimen for a liver/small-bowel graft, it is important to take as long a length of thoracic aorta as possible, and also to leave a stump of aorta distal to the superior mesenteric artery so that this area can be closed safely. The preparation of the liver/small-bowel graft on the back table primarily involves the thoracic aorta and ligating the numerous intercostal branches. Typically, the pancreas distal to the left of the portal vein is removed, and this edge of the pancreas is then oversewn with a nonabsorbable monofilament suture. The distal end of the aorta just distal to the superior mesenteric artery is also oversewn.

Preparation of the recipient for implantation includes central venous access, arterial monitoring, and multiple peripheral venous access. It is also impor-

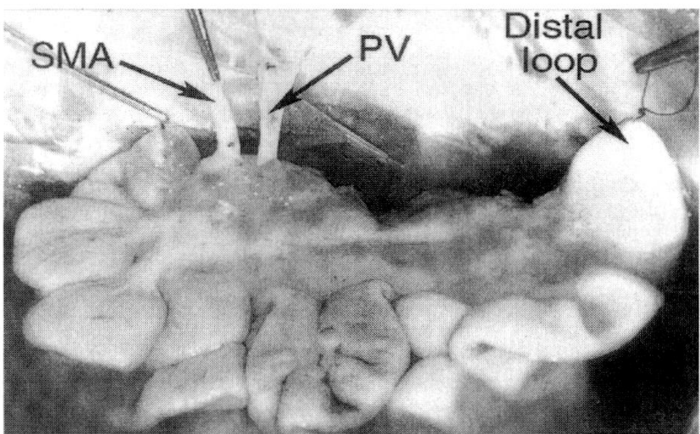

FIG. 1. Second table: small bowel graft. The superior mesenteric artery and superior mesenteric vein have been skeletonized. The distal end of the bowel is marked with a tie to ensure proper positioning in the recipient. *PV*, portal vein; *SMA*, superior mesenteric artery

tant to monitor the body temperature closely. For a patient undergoing isolated small-bowel transplantation, the incision typically depends on previous abdominal incisions. The vast majority of these patients have had numerous operations, and lysis of adhesions will be required. Following this, the retroperitoneum is exposed along the section of the aorta and vena cava. The superior mesenteric artery of the isolated small-bowel graft is then anastomosed to the recipient infrarenal aorta. The venous drainage can be systemic or portal. Systemic drainage is preferred whenever liver disease is present or when previous surgeries make an anastomosis to the splanchnic venous system impossible. The venous anastomosis to the interior vena cava should be located somewhat more cephalad than the level of the arterial one. Extreme care should be taken to avoid twisting the vessels. Intestinal continuity is then restored typically between the recipient's duodenum and the jejunum of the allograft. An ileocolostomy is then created, and finally a loop ileostomy is brought up to the skin to help monitor graft function and to facilitate biopsies.

The surgical technique for liver/small-bowel transplantation has evolved over the past 5 years (Fig. 2) [6]. The technique we routinely use today leaves the hilar structures of the liver undisturbed, retaining the hepatic duodenal biliary system intact. We believe that there are numerous advantages to this approach, including limited second-table dissection, prevention of torsion about the portal vein after implantation, and eliminating the need for biliary tract reconstruction. The liver/small-bowel graft is then implanted orthotopically in a similar way to liver transplantation. The suprahepatic vena caval anastomosis is completed first, followed by the infrahepatic vena cava. Typically, the aortic conduit of the graft is anastomosed to the supraceliac aorta of the recipient. A decision on whether to remove the patient's native abdominal organs is dependent on their functional status. Typically, for patients who have motility disorders such as intestinal pseudoobstruction, all of the abdominal viscera are removed with the exception of the proximal stomach and distal colon. For those patients who have more typical causes of short-bowel syndrome, and have a functioning proximal GI tract, this will remain intact. If the native stomach, duodenum, pancreas, and spleen are left in place, venous drainage of the native portal system is facilitated by the creation of a porta caval shunt at some point during the transplantation procedure. We typically create this shunt following reperfusion of the allograft, although it can be done earlier.

After transplantation, regardless of whether the patient has received a liver/small-bowel or an isolated small-bowel transplantation, immune suppression consists of induction therapy with basiliximab, followed by maintenance therapy with tacrolimus and steroids. Numerous other agents are given in the perioperative period, including for antiviral, antibacterial, and antifungal agents.

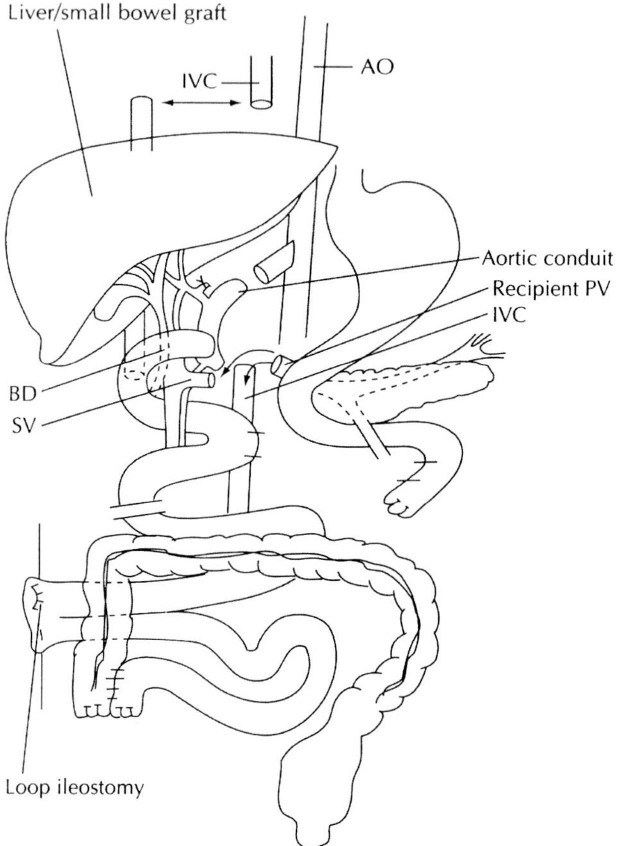

FIG. 2. Transplantation of the combined liver/small-bowel graft. *AO*, aorta; *BD*, bile duct; *IVC*, inferior vena cava; *SV*; splenic vein

Posttransplantation, the most difficult problem for these patients is the development of rejection. Rejection is diagnosed following endoscopic biopsy of the allograft. Endoscopy and biopsy are carried out by protocol twice a week for the first 6 weeks, and thereafter when clinically indicated. Typical clinical findings include diarrhea, abdominal pain, and distension. Histologically, the diagnosis of rejection is made with the findings of mild cryptitis, inflammatory infiltrate in the lamina propria, and apoptosis of crypt cells [8]. Rejection episodes can be treated with steroid boluses or an antilymphocyte preparation, or for refractory rejection with explantation of the allograft.

We initiated an Intestinal Transplant Program at the University of Nebraska Medical Center in 1990. During that time, we have evaluated over 250 patients for some form of intestinal transplantation procedure. From October 1990 through April 2001, we performed 117 intestinal transplants in 106 patients.

Seventy-four of these transplants were liver/small-bowel procedures. Of these 74 liver/small-bowel transplantations, 5 were performed under cyclosporine immune suppression, and 61 under tacrolimus immune suppression. Eight of these patients had undergone some form of prior transplantation. Beginning in December 1994, we initiated an isolated small-bowel transplantation program [9]. Since that time, we have performed 43 isolated intestinal transplants. The causes of intestinal failure are listed in Table 1 [10]. The clinical activity of our intestinal transplantation program is depicted in Fig. 3.

Most of the 117 intestinal transplantations performed were in children (Table 2) [10]. Overall, the children undergoing liver/small-bowel transplantation were considerably younger than those undergoing isolated small-bowel

TABLE 1. Cause of intestinal failure ($n = 106$)

	LSB	ISB
Midgut volvulus	15	10
Gastroschisis	13	3
Intestinal atresia	9	2
Necrotizing enterocolitis	8	3
Hirschsprung disease	8	1
Pseudoobstruction	6	8
Massive gut resection	4	5
Microvillus inclusion	3	3
Others	3	2

LSB, liver/small bowel; ISB, isolated small bowel

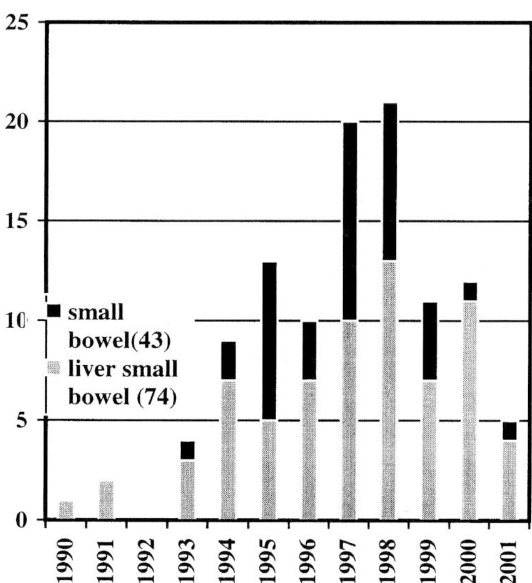

FIG. 3. Intestinal transplantations 1990 to 2001 ($n = 117$)

TABLE 2. Recipient demographics ($n = 117$ transplantations)

	LSB	ISB
Pediatric cases	69	35
Adult cases	5	8
Mean age pediatric cases	2.8 years	6 years
Mean age adult cases	30 years	35 years
Indication for transplantation		
Liver disease	74 (1 case with BA)	15
Sepsis		14
Loss of access		9
Other		5
UNOS status (liver)	1-23, 2A-1, 2B-31, 3-19	NA
Previous transplants	9 (1 LSB, 5 ISB, 3 L)	7 (5 ISB, 1 L, 1 LSB)

LSB, liver/small bowel; ISB, isolated small bowel; BA, biliary atresia; UNOS, United Network for Organ Sharing; NA, not applicable; L, liver

transplantation. The indications for intestinal transplantation were TPN liver disease in all but one patient receiving liver/small-bowel transplantation. For isolated small-bowel transplantation, the indications included liver disease, sepsis, loss of venous access, and other causes. Of the 74 liver/small-bowel transplants, 24 patients were in the ICU at the time of transplantation, another 31 were hospitalized but outside the ICU, and only 19 were at home prior to transplantation. A previous transplantation had been performed in 9 of the liver/small-bowel transplantation patients and 7 of the isolated small-bowel transplant patients (Table 2). The donors were selected based on a variety of factors. In particular, these included hemodynamic stability, suitable laboratory tests for liver and renal function, and negative serologies. We made every attempt to use donors who were smaller than the potential recipients. The details of the donor selection criteria are given in Table 3. Cross-match data were only available in a retrospective manner. We attempted to keep the cold ischemia time as short as possible, with 12h being our upper limit of acceptability.

The surgical procedures performed at the University of Nebraska Medical Center were detailed above. The liver/small-bowel operative technique has evolved. The old technique was performed in only the first 5 patients. Following this, the remaining 69 patients received the en bloc surgical procedure. In 11 of these patients, the liver/small-bowel transplantation procedure was associated with an evisceration of abdominal organs. For the isolated small-bowel transplants, 18 patients underwent portal drainage. However, if there was evidence of underlying liver disease, or if the vascular anatomy was not suitable, then drainage of these isolated/small-bowel allografts was directed into the inferior vena cava. This was performed in the remaining 25 patients.

TABLE 3. Donor information

	Pediatric	Adult
Liver/small bowel		
Mean age	0.3 years	9.1 years
Mean weight	17 lb	66 lb
Donor/Recipient ratio	0.7 (.3–1)	0.9 (.45–2)
Mean cold ischemia time	10.6 h (7.8–16 h)	—
Isolated		
Mean age	2.1 years	10.7 years
Mean weight	22 lb	77 lb
Donor/Recipient ratio	0.6 (.4–1.2)	0.6 (.4–.9)
Mean cold ischemia time	9 h (7–13.5 h)	—

Ranges are shown in parentheses

Postoperative immune suppression consisted of cyclosporine in the first 5 patients. Following that, the remaining 112 transplants were performed with tacrolimus immune suppression. More recently, in the last 26 patients we have added basiliximab. In 11 patients we also added sirolimus to preserve renal function.

We have analyzed our experience with primary intestinal transplantation with tacrolimus-based immune suppression. This covered 97 patients. The vast majority of patients had at least one rejection episode. The time of the first rejection episode was typically within about the first 2 weeks. At least 80% of the patients had their first episode of rejection in the first posttransplantation year. Treatment typically consisted of steroid boluses initially. However, an antilymphocyte preparation was required in 24 of the 97 patients, and explantation of six isolated small-bowel allografts and 1 liver/small-bowel allograft was required owing to severe rejection. We have recently added basiliximab as induction therapy to help reduce instances of rejection. The results of this experience are given in Table 3.

In summary, we have seen a significant reduction in the number of small-bowel rejection episodes. We have also noted a significant decrease in fungal infections, which is probably related to the decreased need for antirejection therapy. However, the length of hospitalization has not changed. Surgical complications are relatively common and occurred in 66% of the liver/small-bowel transplant operations and 45% of the isolated small-bowel operations. The most common indications for reoperation were related to intraabdominal sepsis. These included bowel perforation, intestinal leaks, and abscesses. Vascular complications were relatively uncommon, but there were two arterial thromboses in the liver/small-bowel and one in the isolated small-bowel transplant group. There was an episode of portal vein thrombosis in each of the isolated and liver/small-bowel transplantation groups.

Infectious complications were also relatively common. Bacterial infections were identified in 93% of the patients following transplantation. The site of the isolates included blood, peritoneum, central line and lungs. The most common pathogens included *Pseudomonas*, *Klebsiella*, and *Escherichia coli*. Vancomycin-resistant *Enterococcus faecium* was cultured in 14 patients. Fungal infections were identified in 25% of the patients, with the majority of them being *Candida* species.

CMV infections have been identified as a significant source of morbidity in intestinal transplant recipients [11]. We diagnosed CMV infections in 16 of our patients. The site of the CMV infections included the small bowel (10), lung (4), and blood (2). There was only one death due to CMV. Adenovirus was cultured in 43 patients. It is most commonly cultured from the small bowel. Fortunately, there were only two deaths in this group of patients, both the result of adenovirus pneumonia.

Lymphoproliferative disease was diagnosed in a total of 9 patients. The median time to diagnosis was approximately 4 months. The sites of diagnosis included tonsils/adenoids (3), lung or mediastinum (2), GI tract (2), and peripheral lymph nodes (2). Initially we treated these patients with reduced immune suppression. However, this resulted in the catastrophic loss of small-bowel allografts in the liver/small-bowel transplant recipients. Subsequently, we have initiated a trial of low-dose cyclophosphamide and reduced immune suppression in 8 patients [12]. Of the nine patients with lymphoproliferative disease, 4 are disease-free with functioning allografts (1 isolated small bowel, 3 liver/small bowel). Two of the isolated small-bowel transplant recipients had their grafts explanted, with one of these patients now being successfully retransplanted. Three other liver/small-bowel transplant recipients died.

Survival after intestinal transplantation is shown in Fig. 4. As can be seen, the isolated small-bowel transplant group has done the best. This has been because we are able to remove the allograft to save the patient's life. The causes of death are primarily sepsis related in both liver/small-bowel and isolated small-bowel groups. Other causes include some vascular catastrophe in four of the liver/small bowel-transplant patients. Two patients died at home suddenly and without a known cause.

In the isolated small-bowel transplant group there were 18 isolated small-bowel grafts that had to be removed. The most common reason for this was some form of rejection. There were two technical losses, including one arterial and one portal vein thrombosis. Two patients lost their grafts owing to a reduction in immune suppression due to posttransplant lymphopraliferative disorder. Three patients died with functioning grafts. Chronic rejection was diagnosed in two patients following explantation.

The goal of intestinal transplantation is not only to prevent and eliminate life-threatening complications of TPN, but also to provide nutritional

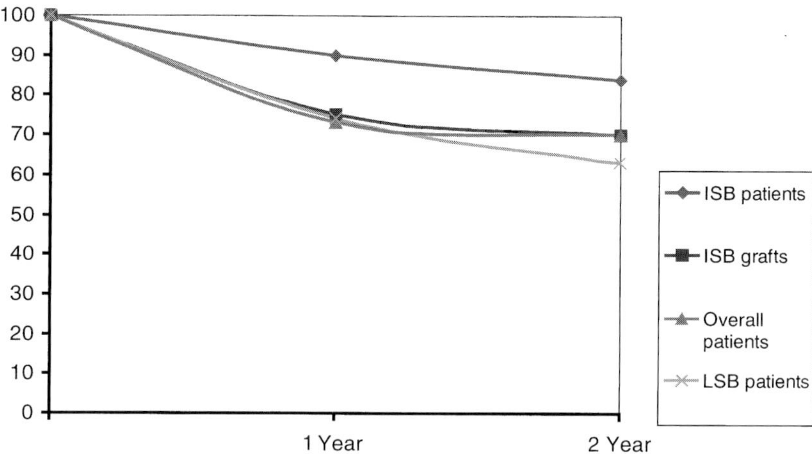

FIG. 4. Survival after intestinal transplantation

independence for these patients. For recipients of both liver and liver/ small-bowel transplantation, the median time to discontinuing TPN and receiving a full enteral diet was approximately 2 months. Virtually every patient who survived and had an intact allograft was able to discontinue TPN, although many required enteral feeding via a feeding tube. This is particularly true for many of the young children who had developed a food aversion. The median length of stay in hospital for these patients was 54 days. The average median cost of an intestinal transplant with or without liver was approximately \$275 000. Several insurance companies pay for intestinal transplantation. The most recent addition to this list is the United States Federal Government.

In summary, intestinal transplantation has become an effective life-saving procedure for patients with life-threatening complications of intestinal failure. The surgical techniques have been refined. We now know that the short-term survival is satisfactory, but we still await the long-term results. We have made substantial inroads into the management of rejection episodes, but while intestinal transplantation has become successful, the costs and length of stay in hospital are still too high. The first 10 years of carrying out intestinal transplantations have been exciting, and we have seen great improvements. Hopefully, over the next 10 years we can improve the results to the point where they are similar to those of renal transplantation.

References

1. HCFA (2001) Health Care Financing Administration Division of Integrated Delivery Systems. List of Medicare-approved intestinal transplant centers. www.hcfa.gov/medicare/intstnlist.htm

2. Howard L, Ament M, Fleming CR, et al. (1995) Current use and clinical outcome of home parenteral and enteral nutrition therapies in the United States. Gastroenterology 109:355–365
3. Kelly D (1998) Liver complications of pediatric parenteral nutrition—epidemiology. Nutrition 14:153–157
4. Kaufman S, Atkinson J, Bianchi A, et al. (2001) Indications for pediatric intestinal transplantation: a position paper of the American Society of Transplantation. Pediatr Transplant 5:80–87
5. Sindhi R, Landmark J, Shaw B Jr, et al. (1996) Combined liver/small bowel transplantation using a blood group compatible but nonidentical donor. Transplantation 61: 1782–1783
6. DeRoover A, Langnas A (1998) Surgical methods of small bowel transplantation. Curr Opin Organ Transplant 4:335–342
7. Iyer K, Kaufman S, Sudan D, et al. (2001) Long-term results of intestinal tranpslantation for pseudo-obstruction in children. J Pediatr Surg 36:174–177
8. Lee R, Nakamura K, Tsamandas A, et al. (1996) Pathology of human intestinal transplantation. Gastroenterology 110:1820–1834
9. Sudan D, Kaufman S, Shaw B, et al. (2000) Isolated intestinal transplantation for intestinal failure. Am J Gastroenterol 95:1506–1515
10. Langnas A, Chinnakotla S, Sudan D, et al. (2001) Ten Year Experience with Intestinal Transplantation. American Journal of Transplantation In press
11. Manez R, Kusne S, Green M, et al. (1995) Incidence and risk factors associated with the development of cytomegalovirus disease after intestinal transplantation. Transplantation 59:1010–1014
12. Gross T, Hinrichs S, Winner J, et al. (1998) Treatment of post-transplant lymphoproliferative disease (PTLD) following solid organ transplantation with low-dose chemotherapy. Ann Oncol 9:339–340

Clinical Experience of Small Bowel/Multivisceral Transplantation at the University of Miami

Seigo Nishida, Tomoaki Kato, David Levi, Jose R. Nery, Naveen Mittal, Juan Madariaga, and Andreas G. Tzakis

Summary. Some patients with intestinal failure have life-threatening total parenteral nutrition (TPN) complications. Intestinal transplantation is the lifesaving alternative for these patients. We reviewed 95 consecutive intestinal transplants performed between December 1994 and November 2000 at the University of Miami. Fifty-four cases were pediatric and 41 cases were adult. Forty-nine patients were men and 46 women. The causes of intestinal failure were mesenteric thrombosis ($n = 12$), necrotizing enterocolitis ($n = 11$), gastroschisis ($n = 11$), voluvulus ($n = 9$), desmoid tumor ($n = 8$), intestinal atresia ($n = 6$), trauma ($n = 5$), Hirschsprung's disease ($n = 5$), Crohn's disease (n = 5), pseudoobstruction ($n = 4$), and other ($n = 19$). All patients had TPN-related complications, and 67 patients had liver failure. Isolated intestinal transplantation was performed in 27 cases. Liver and intestinal transplantation was performed in 28 cases. Multivisceral transplantation was performed in 40 cases. Mean cold ischemic time was 480 ± 12.3 min. The 1-year patient and graft survival rates of isolated intestinal transplantation since 1998 were 84% and 72%, respectively. Since 1998, we have been using a zoom videoendoscope and induction with daclizumab. The 1-year patient and graft survivals of isolated intestinal transplants before 1998 were 75% and 68%, respectively. The 1-year patient and graft survival rates of liver and intestinal transplantation were 40% and 37%, respectively. The 1-year patient and graft survival rates of multivisceral transplantation were 48% and 40%, respectively. The causes of death were sepsis after rejection ($n = 14$). respiratory failure ($n = 8$), sepsis ($n = 6$), multiple organ failure ($n = 4$), arterial graft infection ($n = 3$), aspergillosis ($n = 2$), post transplant lymphoproliferative dis-

Division of Transplantation, Department of Surgery, University of Miami, Highland Professional Building, Suite 514, 1801 NW 9th Avenue, Miami, FL 33136, USA

orders ($n = 2$), intracranial bleeding ($n = 2$), fungemia ($n = 1$), chronic rejection ($n = 1$), graft-versus-host disease ($n = 1$), necrotizing enterocolitis ($n = 1$), pancreatitis ($n = 1$), pulmonary embolism ($n = 1$), and viral encephalitis ($n = 1$). Intestinal transplantation provided a lifesaving alternative for patients with intestinal failure. Patient and graft survival rates following isolated intestinal transplantation were better than those after liver–intestinal transplantation and multivisceral transplantation. The prognosis is better when the transplant is performed prior to the onset of liver failure.

Key words. Small bowel transplantation, Multivisceral transplantation, Intestinal failure

Introduction

Intestinal transplantation has been developed for some patients with intestinal failure who have life-threatening total parenteral nutrition (TPN) complications. Intestinal transplantation is the life-saving alternative for these patients. Alexis Carrel performed an experimental intestinal transplantation in 1902 [1]. Lillehei et al. reported a functioning autotransplanted intestine after cold preservation in 1959 [2]. Starzl and Kaupp carried out a polysplanchnic transplantation in 1960 [3]. Clinical intestinal transplantations were performed in the 1960s, but the rejection and infection rates were insurmountable barriers for a long time. In 1988, Grant et al. reported a successful intestinal transplantation in a pig using cyclosporine [4], and Goulet et al. in Paris and Deltz et al. in Kiel reported the successful intestinal transplantations shortly afterward [5, 6]. Grant et al. in Ontario reported the first successful liver–intestinal transplantation with cyclosporine in 1990 [7], and Todo et al. in Pittsburgh, developed the intestinal transplantation with tacrolimus in the early 1990s [8]. Intestinal and multivisceral transplantation at the University of Miami was started in 1994. By November 2000, we had performed 95 intestinal transplantations, including 27 isolated intestinal transplantations, 28 liver–intestinal transplantations, and 40 multivisceral transplantations. The surgical techniques, rejection monitoring, and cytomegalovirus prophylaxis have evolved over the years. We present our clinical experience of intestinal and multivisceral transplantation. We review 95 consecutive intestinal transplantations performed at the University of Miami. All the data were collected by chart review retrospectively. Patient and graft survival estimates were obtained using the Kaplan–Meier product limit method. The log–rank test was performed for survival analysis.

Demographics of the Recipients and Donors

A total of 95 transplantations were performed in 87 patients. The number of transplantations per year has increased since 1994 (Fig. 1). The sex distribution was approximately equal, with 49 male patients (52%) and 46 female patients (48%). There were 54 pediatric patients (57%) and 41 adult patients (43%). The age distributions of the pediatric and adult recipients are shown in Figs. 2 and 3. Most of the pediatric cases were less than 5 years old, and the oldest recipient was 53 years old. The types of transplantation were: 27 cases of isolated intestinal transplantation (28%), 28 cases of combined liver and intestinal transplantation (29%), and 40 cases of multivisceral transplantation, including the stomach, pancreas, intestine and/or liver (43%) (Fig. 4). All

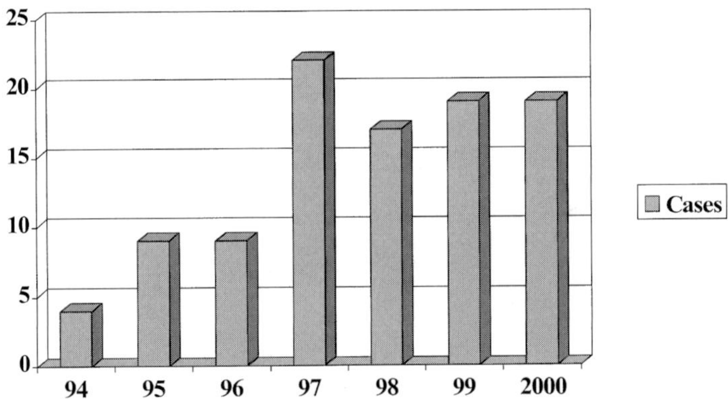

Fig. 1. Number of intestinal tranplants

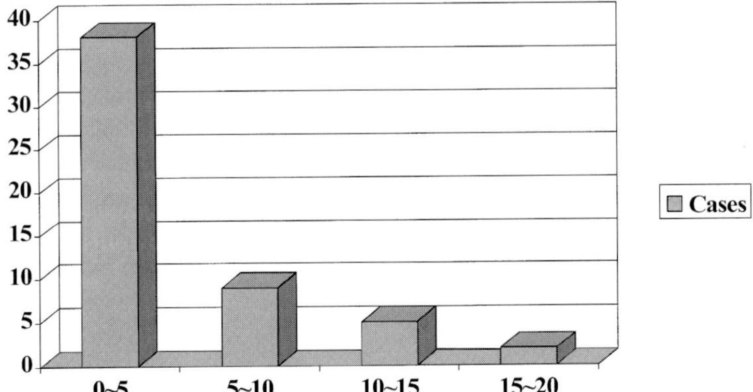

Fig. 2. Age of pediatric recipients

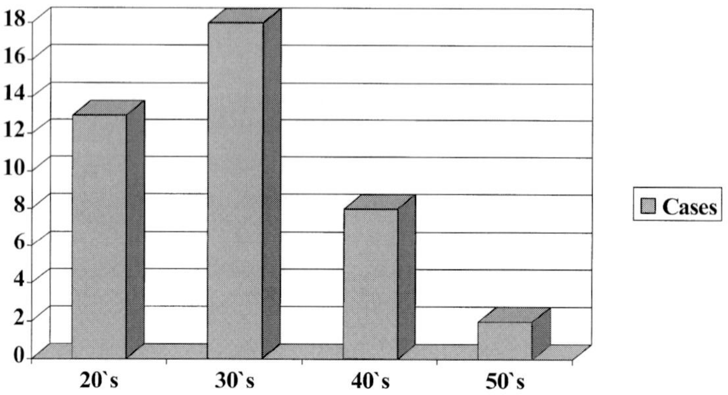

FIG. 3. Age of adult recipients

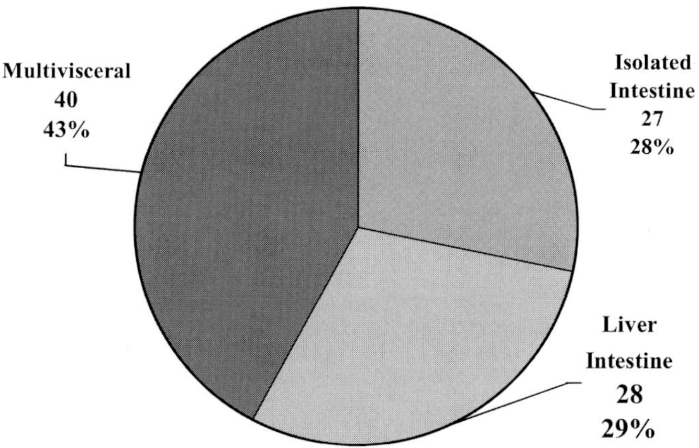

FIG. 4. Type of transplantation

the grafts were obtained from a cadaveric donor. There were 56 male donors (59%) and 39 female donors (41%). The age distribution of the donors is shown in Fig. 5. The donor selection criteria were: identical blood type; the same or smaller body weight if possible; and serology negative except for cytomegalovirus (CMV).

Before organ procurement, all the teams, including liver transplant team, kidney transplant team, pancreas transplant team, and intestinal transplant team, need to consider the anatomy of the donor and reach an agreement on how the organs should be divided.

To procure the organs, the portal vein is cut above the splenic vein confluence, and the superior mesenteric artery is cut with the aortic cuff in the case of a normal isolated intestinal transplant. If a right replaced hepatic

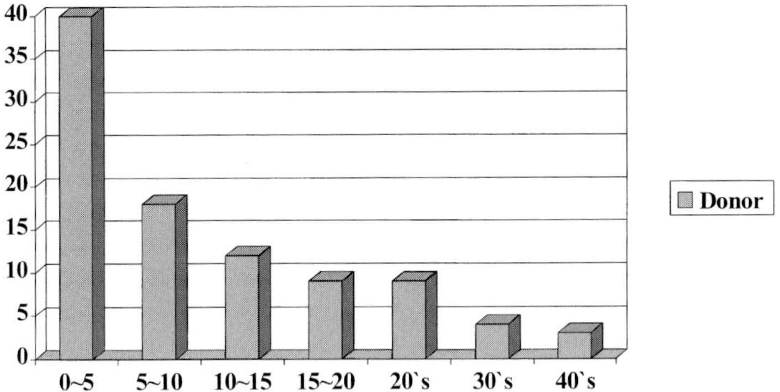

FIG. 5. Age of donors

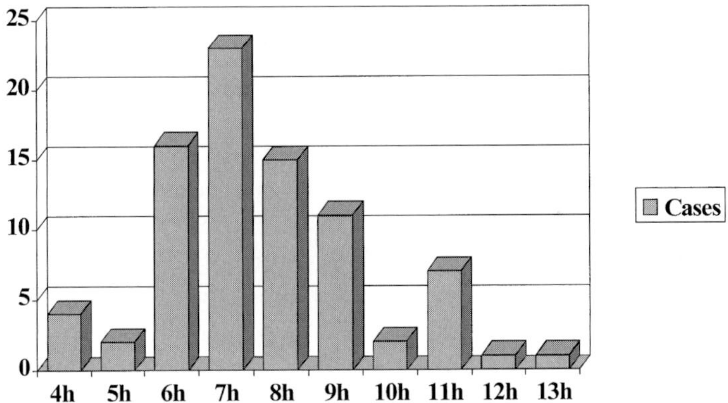

FIG. 6. Cold ischemic time

artery exists, the superior mesenteric artery is cut distal to the replaced hepatic artery. Both the celiac and superior mesenteric arteries are procured, with the thoracic and abdominal aorta above the renal artery in a multivisceral transplantation. The cold ischemic time should be minimized as much as possible to prevent graft injury. The graft is then flushed with cold University of Wisconsin (UW) solution. Our mean cold ischemic time was 480 ± 12.3 min. The longest cold ischemic time was 13 h. The cold ischemic time distribution is shown in Fig. 6.

Indications and Patient Evaluation

The indications for intestinal transplantation are intestinal failure, patients with life-threatening total parenteral nutrition complications, including liver failure, and central vein access difficulty due to thrombosis. Most intestinal

TABLE 1. Cause of intestinal failure

Mesenteric thrombosis	12
Necrotizing enterocolitis	11
Gastroschisis	11
Volvulus	9
Desmoid tumor	8
Intestinal atresia	6
Trauma	5
Hirschsprung's disease	5
Crohn's disease	5
Pseudoobstruction	4
Others	19

failure patients do well on parenteral nutrition. However, some patients cannot tolerate parenteral nutrition owing to life-threatening complications. The causes of intestinal failure were mesenteric thrombosis, necrotizing enterocolitis, gastroschisis, volvulus, desmoid tumor, intestinal atresia, trauma, Hirschsprung's disease, Crohn's disease, pseudoobstruction, and others. The causes of the intestinal failures are given in Table 1. All patients had TPN-related complications, and 67 patients had liver failure.

Potential candidates for intestinal transplantation require careful assessment, including early referral, a detailed history of TPN, a detailed medical history, a detailed surgical history, and radiographic images of their gastrointestinal anatomy and vascular access. Precise information regarding all types of previous surgery and the length of the intestinal remnant is very important. The liver function test needs to be evaluated carefully. Some patients will need a liver biopsy to confirm the level of liver injury. If irreversible liver injury exists, a transplantation including the liver needs to be considered. Kidney evaluation is also important, because some patients already have kidney failure or a borderline kidney function due to a very complicated medical and surgical history. In addition to that, baseline immunosupression, e.g., with tacrolimus, has side effects which relate to kidney function.

Recipient Operation

We performed three types of operation (see Fig. 4). Isolated intestinal transplantation includes only the small intestine. The arterial anastomosis is usually performed between the superior mesenteric artery of the donor and the aorta of the recipient with the interposition of a jump graft of the donor iliac, carotid, or thoracic artery. The arterial graft can be anastomosed to the supraceliac or infrarenal aorta of the recipient. In some cases, the superior mesenteric artery (SMA) can be anastomosed directly end-to-end to the aorta or the SMA of the recipient. Portal vein anastomosis is performed in two ways. One is portal drainage, the other is systemic drainage. In portal drainage, the portal vein is anastomosed end-to-end to the recipient's superior mesenteric vein (SMV), the confluence of the SMV and the splenic vein, or the side of the portal vein.

If the desired procedure is technically difficult, systemic drainage is performed. The portal vein is anastomosed to the inferior cava in an end-to-side manner. Our data show no difference in the metabolic and immunological results between portal drainage and systemic drainage.

Combined liver and intestinal transplantation includes the liver and the intestine as a composite graft. The arterial anastomosis is usually performed in an end-to-side manner between the donor's aorta and recipient aorta with the interposition of an aortic graft. Caval anastomoses are usually performed in an end-to-side manner with a suprahepatic caval anstomosis for venous outflow (piggyback technique).

Multivisceral transplantation includes the intestine, stomach, pancreas, and/or liver with or without the kidney. The arterial anastomosis and the caval anastomosis are the same as for the combined liver and intestinal transplantation. The proximal end of the intestine in an isolated intestinal or a combined liver and intestine transplantation is usually anastomosed side-to-side to the recipient intestine. In multivisceral transplantation, the proximal anastomosis is performed between the donor stomach and the recipient esophagus. A tube-feeding catheter is usually placed from the jejunum or the stomach. The distal end of the intestine is usually exteriorized as a stoma to decompress the bowel, and is used for rejection monitoring. If a remnant colon exists, we usually perform the anstomosis between the colon and the distal part of the intestinal graft.

If the size of the donor intestine or liver is larger than the size of the re-cipient abdominal cavity, we perform a resection of the intestine or liver. If the graft size is larger than the recipient abdominal cavity, abdominal closure may require a mesh or staged approximation. A skin flap, muscle flap, or syn-thetic mesh is used for cases where there is a size discrepancy.

Postoperative Management

After intestinal transplantation, patients require intensive postoperative mon-itoring. This includes hemodynamic monitoring with a Swan-Ganz catheter, arterial blood pressure, central venous pressure, pulmonary capillary wedge pressure, oxygen saturation, heart rate, respiratory rate, body temperature, urinary output, abdominal drainage output, and ostomy output. Fluid replacement is usually necessary; patients have a tendency to be hypovolemic due to fluid loss and a high ostomy output. An adequate volume of fluid is essential until the patient starts to mobilize fluid.

Ventilator support at this period is very important because the fluid balance of the patient is usually positive and the lungs are wet. Until the patients starts to mobilize fluid, ventilator support should have a positive end-expiratory pressure. Baseline immunosuppression is usually with tacrolimus and a steroid. Tacrolimus is maintained at the high level of 15–20 ng/ml, with parenteral or enteral administration. Steroids are administrated by bolus for an intense course after the transplantation and at a maintenance dose thereafter.

Daclizumab (Zenapax) is used for induction therapy. Rapamycin (Sirolimus) is used for patients who have shown persistent rejection or complications from Tacrolimus, such as kidney failure or seizure. Some patients had a low combined dose regimen of tacrolimus and rapamycin. Campath is another ongoing regimen which is sometimes used.

Prophylaxis against CMV is essential. We have started using a new regimen of anti-CMV immunoglobulin (CytoGam). CytoGam is administered at 100 mg/kg every other day i.v. for 1 month, and then every 2 weeks for 3 months together with intravenous ganciclovir. Since we started this anti-CMV protocol, we have not experienced any severe CMV infection. We have also used CMV-positive donors safely. An antifungal such as amphotericin B and broad-spectrum antibiotics are essential in the immediate postoperation period. A proton pump inhibitor, and gut decontamination with amphotericin B, gentamycin, and kanamycin are also carried out.

Enteral feeding via a feeding tube is usually started 4–6 days after transplantation to maintain mucosal function. An elemental diet such as Vivonex is initiated at a reduced strength and low dose. If the intestine functions well, tube feeding is slowly increased until the ideal level in reached, and maintained. Oral intake is started after 2 weeks if the patient's intestine continues to function well. TPN is slowly tapered off if the patient can get sufficient calories from tube feeding or by oral intake. Patients are usually on TPN for a long time. We must pay special attention to the fluid balance when tapering off the TPN.

Rejection monitoring starts on postoperative day 3. We use endoscopy and biopsies for rejection monitoring. Zoom videoendoscopy was carried out twice a week for 1 month, once a week for 3 months, every day, or every other day to monitor the ongoing pathology [9]. Since we started this protocol, we have often avoided delays in the treatment of rejection and prevented over-immunosuppression. Clinical signs of rejection, such as high output, diarrhea, and fever, are also very important. If there is any suspicion of rejection, we do a biopsy of the intestine.

Complications

Rejection

Rejection is a major problem after intestinal transplantation. The clinical signs of rejection are fever, diarrhea, high output, motility problems, and abdominal pain. Delays in the diagnosis of rejection are usually critical for the patient. We started a protocol using zoom videoendoscopy because of the real danger of rejection. As mentioned above, we performed endoscopy twice a week for 1 month, once a week for 3 months, every day, or every other day to monitor the ongoing pathology. The endoscopic film is analyzed for the height of the villi, shape of the tips of the villi, background erythema, bleeding in the villi, and friability of the mucosa. We have used a scoring system for the probability of rejection, and an ongoing investigation of the rejection monitoring system. Some patients showing moderate rejection have recovered with immunosuppression. However, all cases of severe rejection have resulted in a lost the graft. A steroid bolus and a course of steroids are used to treat rejection. Rapamycin is added for persistent rejection under a tacrolimus regimen. Tacrolimus is maintained at a level of more than 20 ng/ml. OKT 3 is administered for episodes of rejection which do not respond to steroids.

Infections

Infection is another major problem after intestinal transplantation. We have experience of line infection, wound infection, intraabdominal abscess, pneumonia, urinary tract infection, sepsis after rejection, fugal infection, and viral infection. After rejection, bacterial translocation tends to occur and sepsis continues. Gram-negative infection is frequently observed. If patients are overimmunosuppressed, sepsis can occur very easily. The balance of the immunosuppression is the most important aspect of the management of intestinal transplant patients. The patient will have many lines inside the body, such as a central line, arterial line, urinary catheter, chest tube, and abdominal drainage. All the lines need to be monitored and cultured frequently. If a line is not absolutely essential, it should be removed as soon as possible to prevent it becoming a cause of sepsis. The most common bacteria are *Escherichia coli, Enterococcus faecium, Staphylococcus, Klebsiella, Proteus, Pseudomonas aeruginosa*, and *Enterobacter cloacae* [10]. Fugal infections are also common, such as *Aspergillus* and *Candida*. Viral infections are mainly cause by cytomegalovirus and Epstein–Barr virus (EBV). Diagnostic tests for CMV and EBV are performed by polymerase chain reaction (PCR). Prophylaxis with ganciclovir and CytoGam has decreased the number of cases of CMV infection. EBV infection is related to PTLD. PTLD is also treated with ganciclovir and CytoGam. Adenovirus infection is very serious for pediatric patients, since it can causes critical pneumonia and enteritis. Respiratory syncytial virus (RSV) infection also cause critical pneumonia in pediatric patients. The treatment is ribavirin and a reduction of immunosuppression.

Surgical Complications

We had three cases of arterial graft infection. The graft ruptured after the infection, and the patient died suddenly. Careful attention is paid to aseptic procedures during the operation and in donor procurement, and large amounts of antibiotic solution are applied after the vascular anastomosis and before the abdominal closure. Intestinal anstomosis leakages also occur. Esophagogastrostomies were reanastomosed and ileocolic anstomoses were conservatively treated. All such cases were controlled, and the patients recovered. Postoperative bleeding after the transplantation occurred in a patient who had liver dysfunction and a low platelet count. All the patients were taken back to the operating room and hemostases were performed surgically. Meticulous hemostasis is essential for patients with a history of multiple surgery, and for borderline liver-function patients.

Renal Failure

Some patient had borderline kidney function before the transplantation, and some experienced renal failure after transplantation. They were treated with CVVHD, hemodialysis (HD), or kidney transplantation. Antibiotics, antifungicides, and antiviral medication have side effects on renal function, as does tacrolimus. A daily evaluation of the medication dose and the involvement of a nephrologist are essential in the management of such critically ill patients.

Survival

The 1-year patient and graft survival rates of isolated intestinal transplantation since 1998 were 84% and 72%, respectively (Fig. 7). Since 1998, we have been using a zoom videoendoscope and induction with daclizumab. Before 1998, the 1-year patient and graft survivals of isolated intestinal transplants were 75% and 68%, respectively. The 1-year patient and graft survivals of liver and intestinal transplantations were 40% and 37%, respectively. The 1-year patient and graft survival rates after multivisceral transplantations were 48% and 40%, respectively. Patient survival rates for each type of transplantion are shown in Fig. 8. Isolated intestinal transplantation without the liver shows a better survival rate than liver–intestinal transplantation or multivisceral transplantation. The prognosis is also better when the transplantation is performed before the onset of liver failure. The causes of death

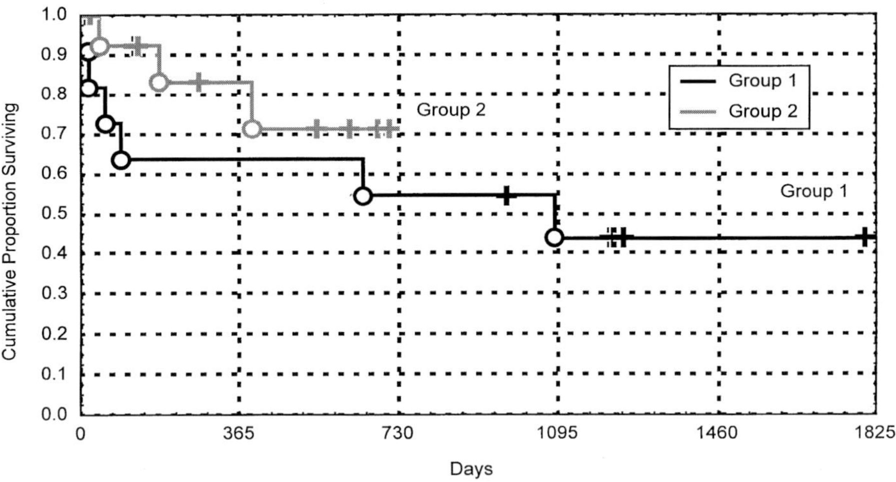

FIG. 7. Patient survival rates (Kaplan–Meier) after isolated intestinal transplantation. Group 1, 1994–1997; Group 2, 1998–2000

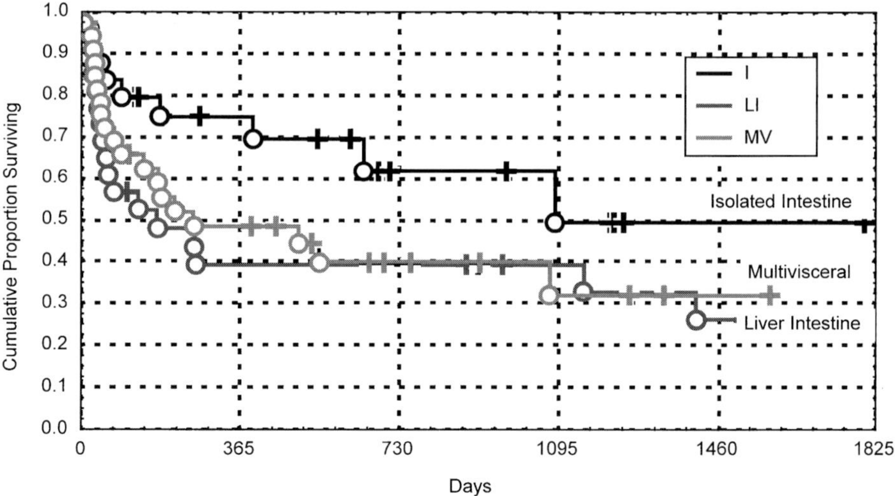

FIG. 8. Patient survival rates (Kaplan–Meier) after three types of transplantation: isolated intestinal; multivisceral; liver–intestine. *Open circles*, complete; *crosses*, censored

were sepsis after rejection ($n = 14$), respiratory failure ($n = 8$), sepsis ($n = 6$), multiple organ failure ($n = 4$), arterial graft infection ($n = 3$), aspergillosis ($n = 2$), PTLD ($n = 2$), intracranial bleeding ($n = 2$), fungemia ($n = 1$), chronic rejection ($n = 1$), graft-versus-host disease ($n = 1$), necrotizing enterocolitis ($n = 1$), pancreatitis ($n = 1$), pulmonary embolism ($n = 1$), and viral encephalitis ($n = 1$).

Evolution

Since 1998, many changes have been made in the field of transplantation; e.g., surgical technique, CMV prophlaxis, zoom videoendoscopy, new immunosuppressive agents, and the prevention of overimmunosuppression.

Systemic drainage to the inferior vena cava is applied, and the results are satisfactory. The metabolic effect and the survival rate are as same as with portal drainage. CMV-positive donors are used safely, with intense CMV prophylaxis by CytoGam. Rejection monitoring with zoom videoendoscopy prevents any delay in the diagnosis of rejection or over immunosuppression. Dacluzimab, rapamycin, and campath are new immunosuppression drugs. These changes have improved the results of intestinal transplantation since 1998. Most patients with successful intestinal transplantation can stop TPN and enjoy excellent rehabilitation. Rejection and infection are still the main problems after intestinal transplantation.

References

1. Carrel A (1902) La technique operatoire des anastomoses vasculaires et la transplantation des visceres. Lyon MEO 98:859
2. Lillehie RC, Goott B, Miller FA (1959) The physiological response of the small bowel of the dog to ischemia, including prolonged in vitro preservation of the small bowel with successful replacement and survival. Ann Surg 150:543–560
3. Starzl TE, Kaupp HA Jr (1960) Mass homotransplantation of abdominal organs in dogs. Surg Forum 11:28–30
4. Grant D, Duff J, Zhong R, et al. (1988) Successful intestinal transplantation in pigs treated with cyclosporine. Transplantation 45:279–284
5. Goulet O, Revillon Y, Canioni D, et al. (1992) Two-and-a-half-year follow-up after isolated small bowel transplant in an infant. Transplant Proc 24:1224–1225
6. Deltz E, Mengel W, Hamelmann H (1990) Small bowel transplantation: report of a clinical case. Progress Pediatr Surg 25:90–96
7. Grant D, Wall W, Mimeault R, et al. (1990) Successful small bowel/liver transplantation. Lancet 335:181–184
8. Todo S, Tzakis A, Abu-Elmagd K, et al. (1994) Current status of intestinal transplantation. Adv Surg 27:295–316
9. Kato T, O'Brien CB, Nishida S, et al. (1999) The first case report of the use of a zoom videoendoscope for the evaluation of small bowel graft mucosa in a human after intestinal transplantation. Gastrointest Endosc 50:257–261
10. Asfar S, Atkinson P, Ghent C, et al. (1996) Small bowel transplantation. A life-saving option for selected patients with intestinal failure. Dig Dis Sci 41:875–583

Intestinal Transplantation at the University of Pittsburgh

J.J. Fung, J. Reyes, N. Murase, G. Bond, and K. Abu-Elmagd

Summary. Until recently, intestinal transplantation had not been as success-ful as other organ transplants. The small bowel is the largest lymphoid organ in the body and is endowed with unique immunological characteristics. Cyclosporine immunosuppression was most often accompanied by a pre-dictable outcome of severe and irreversible rejection, which was associated with a long-term graft function lower than 10%. The advent of tacrolimus in 1990 changed the landscape of intestinal transplantation. The impact of the international adoption of tacrolimus is reflected in single-center reports and the cumulative results of the International Intestinal Transplant Registry, which all show significant improvements in patient and graft survival, and recent 1-year patient survival rates approaching 80%. Based on experimental results from our group, both graft irradiation and bone marrow infusion have been used successfully to reduce the risk of rejection. Recent studies in small and large animals have shown that a small dose of irradiation to the intestine ex vivo does not cause intestinal injury and decreases the risk of acute rejec-tion. Low-dose ex vivo irradiation combined with donor bone marrow has been shown to lead to the effective control of rejection. Although satisfa-ctory results are currently achievable, further improvements in survival and cost-effectiveness are articipated. This could be achieved with early patient referral, proper candidate selection, a better understanding of the graft neuroenteric functions, and new management strategies to overcome some of the immunological and biological barriers that currently challenge intestinal transplant physicians.

Key words. Small-bowel transplantation, Tacrolimus, Short-gut syndrome, Liver transplantation, Multivisceral transplantation

---

Thomas Starzl Transplantation Institute, University of Pittsburgh, 4 Fialk Clinic 3601 5th Avenue, Pittsburgh, PA 15213, USA

Introduction

Intestinal transplantation has recently evolved to become a life-saving procedure for patients with irreversible intestinal failure who can no longer be maintained on total parenteral nutrition (TPN) [1–3]. Irreversible intestinal failure is a requisite condition for intestinal transplant candidacy. The presence of concomitant liver and/or other upper abdominal organ failure dictates the need for extension to either combined liver–intestinal or multivisceral transplantation. The irreversibility of liver failure is determined on the length of liver dysfunction, histological and clinical evidence of cirrhosis, and the possibility of recovery of sufficient functional reserve of the native liver. The three conditions associated with the need for multivisceral transplantation are (a) liver failure associated with extensive thrombosis of the splanchnic venous system, (b) massive gastrointestinal polyposis, and (c) generalized hollow visceral myopathy or neuropathy. Table 1 lists the current indications for intestinal transplantation at the University of Pittsburgh.

The massive lymphoid content and heavy bacterial load of the gut provided formidable barriers to intestinal transplantation in humans until the clinical introduction of tacrolimus in 1989 [4]. After successful preclinical studies, large-scale trials were successfully undertaken at our institution in 1990 [1].

TABLE 1. List of indications for intestinal transplantation at the University of Pittsburgh

Short-gut syndrome
- (a) Necrotizing enterocolitis
- (b) Intestinal atresia
- (c) Midgut volvulus
- (d) Complicated gastroschisis
- (e) Abdominal trauma
- (f) Advanced Crohn's disease
- (g) Extensive surgical adhesions
- (h) Gardener's syndrome (familial polyposis)
- (i) Desmoid tumor
- (j) Mesenteric vascular thrombosis

Defective intestinal motility
- (a) Hollow visceral myopathy
- (b) Total intestinal aganglionosis
- (c) Extensive visceral neuropathy

Impaired enterocyte absorptive function
- (a) Microvillus inclusion disease
- (b) Selective autoimmune enteropathy
- (c) Radiation enteritis
- (d) Massive intestinal polyposis

TABLE 2. Current guidelines for selection of candidates for intestinal transplantation

Recommended criteria
 (1) Age between 6 months and 60 years
 (2) Impending liver failure due to TPN-induced cholestasis
 (3) Premalignant (extensive polyposis) or locally aggressive (desmoid) small-bowel tumors
 (4) Limited venous access
 (5) Frequent line infections with sepsis
 (6) Frequent episodes of severe dehydration despite TPN and fluid supplementation
 (7) Significant limitation in quality of life due to TPN restrictions on daily activities

Relative or absolute contraindications
 (1) Significant, uncorrectable cardiopulmonary insufficiency
 (2) Incurable malignancy
 (3) Persistent systemic infections
 (4) Active hepatitis B infection
 (5) Severe systemic autoimmune disease
 (6) Acquired immune deficiency syndrome

TPN, total parenteral nutrition

Prior to this, worldwide experience in this field had been plagued with a combination of intractable rejection, graft versus host disease, and lethal host infection [2]. Changes in patient selection, the ability to augment tacrolimus-based therapy with newer immunosuppressive agents, and improved medical management of intestinal transplant patients have resulted in significant improvements in patient and graft survival, leading to approval by the United States Health Care Finance Administration to offer intestinal transplantation as a covered medical service in 2000. The guidelines currently recommended for patient selection are shown in Table 2.

Current Results

Intestinal transplantation has been associated with frequent and sometimes severe episodes of allograft rejection. With each rejection episode, intestinal recipients are at high risk of systemic bacterial and fungal sepsis because of the loss of the enteric mucosal functional barrier. This is a significant factor in the morbidity and mortality of intestinal transplantation patients. Tacrolimus and prednisone are routinely administered postoperatively to prevent allograft rejection. Prostaglandin-E$_1$ is added as a renoprotective agent during the early post-transplant period. The induction protocol has changed over time. The interleukin (IL)-2 receptor, high-affinity, α-chain monoclonal antibody daclizumab (Zenapax, Roche Pharmaceuticals) has been used for the past 2 years, with the first dose being given intraoperatively, and four additional weekly doses after transplantation. Only if intestinal rejection becomes difficult to manage, or should tacrolimus toxicity develop, is mycophenolate, mofetil, or rapamycin added to the immunosuppressive regimen. OKT3 or antilymphocyte globulin are reserved for steroid-resistant rejection. With the use of daclizumab, we have noticed a significant reduction in the frequency and severity of acute intestinal allograft rejection. In addition, the application of adjunct immunosuppressive agents have allowed us to lower the relatively high maintenance doses of tacrolimus, thus reducing the incidence of acute and chronic nephrotoxicity, diabetogenicity, and neurotoxicity.

As of March 2001, a total of 166 intestinal transplants have been performed in 155 recipients at our center since May 1990, with a 1-year patient and graft survival of 73% and 69%, respectively, and a 5-year patient and graft survival rate of 52% and 43%, respectively. In the surviving patients, freedom from TPN was the general rule, and over 90% of surviving intestinal transplant recipients are totally enterally maintained. A significant improvement in patient and graft survival has been noted in more recent years (since 1995) compared with earlier results (prior to 1995). The current 1-year patient survival rate is approximately 80%, with a corresponding 1-year graft survival rate of 73% in the second half of our program.

New Developments in Intestinal Transplantation

Based on our earlier experience, it was clear that experimental and clinical research into intestinal transplantation was needed to define a more effective prevention and treatment regimen for acute and chronic rejection. The high incidence of acute cellular rejection, the risk of progression to chronic rejection, and the need for excessive prolonged immunosuppression with its associated infectious and lymphoproliferative complications reinforced the urgent need for a new immunological treatment strategy with a better therapeutic index.

We had previously suggested that persistent multilineage microchimerism is essential for the sustained survival of organ allografts [6, 7]. In addition, we had shown that intestinal leukocytes have inferior tolerogenic qualities [8] due to the mature lymphoid nature of the migratory cells contained within the graft. Thus, we initiated a trial in which ex vivo irradiation of the intestinal component was combined with donor bone marrow (BM) infusion [9]. Radiation was given at doses that eliminated the more mature lymphoid elements from the intestinal allograft without compromising the short- or long-term function of the epithelial or endothelial components of the allograft. By giving the infusion of donor BM cells along with the irradiation of the intestinal graft, we sought to determine whether there would be a reduction in the risk of rejection and the need for chronic heavy immunosuppression, thus increasing patient and graft survival [9, 10].

The preliminary results of this pilot clinical trial of combination graft cytoreduction, adjunct donor BM infusion, and induction therapy with dacluzimab have been encouraging. In our first 14 primary intestinal transplant recipients, with follow-up ranging from 1 to 14 months, the incidence of rejection has been markedly reduced, and no deaths have occurred. One graft was lost from primary nonfunction and was replaced. Whether this experience will lead to a reduction in the risk of graft loss due to chronic rejection, and improve patient survival rates by avoiding the need for heavy immunosuppression will be determined by further follow-up studies. The achievement of these tasks will undoubtedly raise intestinal transplantation to the practical stage, and establish a widely achievable standard of care for patients with end-stage intestinal failure.

Conclusions

The current trends in intestinal transplantation are for improved outcomes, less morbidity, improved resource utilization, and improved quality of life [11]. The latter two considerations are important in assessing the role of small-bowel transplantation compared with other potential therapies. As with kidney transplantation, the use of small-bowel transplantation can be examined on a cost-effectiveness basis owing to the alternative therapy of chronic total parenteral hyperalimentation for patients who do not undergo small-bowel transplantation. Medicare data show that the average yearly cost of TPN in the USA in 1992 was over $150 000, not including the costs of frequent hospitalization, medical equipment, and nursing care. The average cost for small-bowel transplantation is between $200 000 and $250 000, with an average yearly medical cost of $20 000 [12]. As with kidney transplantation, small-bowel transplantation becomes cost-effective by the third year after transplantation. In addition, the recipients of small-bowel transplantation have reported improved quality of life measures compared with TPN dependency [13].

Although satisfactory results are currently achievable, further improvements in limiting morbidity and mortality will lead to improved cost-effectiveness and enhanced survival. This can be achieved with proper patient referral and candidate selection, improved monitoring of allograft function, and new management strategies to overcome some of the immunologic and biologic barriers that currently challenge the intestinal transplant team. If the strategy of combined, the short- and long-term risks of rejection and infection, as well as the continuous need for heavy immunosuppression, should be significantly reduced.

References

1. Abu-Elmagd K, Reyes J, Todo S, et al. (1998) Clinical intestinal transplantation: new perspectives and immunologic considerations. J Am Coll Surg 186:512–527
2. Grant D (1996) International Intestinal Transplant Registry: current results of intestinal transplantation. Lancet 347:1801–1803
3. Todo S, Reyes J, Furukawa H, et al. (1995) Outcome of intestinal transplantation. Ann Surg 222:270–282
4. Abu-Elmagd K, Todo S, Tzakis A, et al. (1994) Three years clinical experience with intestinal transplantation. J Am Coll Surg 179:385–400
5. Abu-Elmagd K, Reyes J, Fung J (1998) Transplantation of the human intestine: the forbidden organ. Curr Opin Organ Transplant 3:286–292
6. Starzl TE, Demetris AJ, Murase N, et al. (1992) Cell migration, chimerism, and graft acceptance. Lancet 339:1579–1582
7. Starzl TE, Demetris AJ, Trucco M, et al. (1993) Cell migration and chimerism after whole-organ transplantation: The basis of graft acceptance. Hepatology 17:1127–1152
8. Murase N, Starzl TE, Tanabe M, et al. (1995) Variable chimerism, graft versus host disease, and tolerance after different kinds of cell and whole-organ transplantation from Lewis to Brown-Norway rats. Transplantation 60:158–171
9. Murase N, Ye Q, Nalesnik MA, et al. (2000) Immunomodulation for intestinal transplantation by allograft irradiation, adjunct donor bone marrow infusion, or both. Transplantation 70:1632–1641
10. Rao AS, Fontes P, Zeevi A, et al. (1995) Augmentation of chimerism in whole-organ recipients by simultaneous infusion of donor bone marrow cells. Transplant Proc 27:210–212
11. Abu-Elmagd K, Reyes J, Fung JJ, et al. (1999) Clinical intestinal transplantation in 1998: Pittsburgh experience. Acta Gastro-Enterol Belg 62:224–247
12. Howard L, Ament M, Fleming R, et al. (1995) Current use and clinical outcome of home parenteral and enteral nutrition therapies in the United States. Gastroenterology 109:355–365
13. DiMartini A, Rovera GM, Graham TO, et al. (1998) Quality of life after small-intestinal transplantation and among home parenteral nutrition patients. J Parenteral Enteral Nutr 22:357–362

Intestinal Transplantation in Children: Experience of a Single Center in Paris

OLIVIER GOULET, DOMINIQUE JAN, FLORENCE LACAILLE,
DANIÈLE CANIONI, JEAN-PIERRE CÉZARD, CLAUDE RICOUR,
and YANN RÉVILLON

Key words. Intestinal transplantation, Children

Introduction

Intestinal transplantation (ITx) has become an alternative for patients with permanent intestinal failure who are dependent on parenteral nutrition (PN) [1]. Our center has been involved in the management of pediatric patients with intestinal failure for a long time. After developing a home PN program [2, 3], we started ITx in 1987 using cyclosporine [4]. One of our earliest patients still survives with a fully functioning graft 12 years later [5]. With the development of FK506 (tacrolimus) in the early 1990s [6], we restarted our ITx program. We now report the results of the largest current European series of consecutive intestinal transplantations in pediatric patients at the Necker-Enfants Malades University Hospital in Paris.

Population and Methods

Between November 1994 and December 2000, 31 children underwent intestinal transplantation. Twelve received isolated intestinal transplantation (ITx), and 19 received combined intestine–liver transplantation (ILTx). There were 9 girls and 22 boys, with an age range of 2.5–15 years (median 5 years). All had been on long-term PN for a median time of 4.5 years (range 18 months to 13 years) for intractable infantile diarrhea ($n = 12$), short bowel syndrome

---

Combined Program of Liver and Intestinal Transplantation, Hôpital Necker-Enfants Malades, 149 rue de Sèvres, 75743 Paris, Cedex 15, France

($n = 9$), long-segment Hirschsprung's disease ($n = 6$), or chronic intestinal pseudoobstruction syndrome ($n = 4$). The patients were selected to receive isolated ITx because of multiple episodes of catheter-related sepsis and/or major vessel thrombosis, or combined liver–ITx (LITx) in cases of liver cirrhosis or severe hepatic fibrosis.

The intestinal grafts were harvested from ABO blood-type-identical cadaveric donors aged between 3 months and 40 years, whose average weight was 23.4 kg (range 5.0–55.0 kg). A lymphocytotoxic cross-match was negative in all patients. Neither donor nor graft pretreatment was performed. Median cold ischemia time, using University of Wisconsin solution, was 6.25 h (range 2–10 h). Small bowel graft length ranged between 1.90 and 4.50 m (median 3.00 m). The right colon was also transplanted in 17 patients. The reconstruction of the gastrointestinal tract included proximal anastomosis of the small bowel graft to the native duodenum or jejunum. The distal end of the graft was exteriorized as stoma.

We used three immunosuppression regimes. 1. Methylprednisolone given as an initial bolus, then at 2 mg/kg/day during the first month, and then tapered to 1 mg/kg/day for 2 months, with a maintenance dose of 0.5 mg/kg/day to the 6th month, and 0.5 mg/kg/every other day at the end of the first year. 2. Tacrolimus (Prograf). Intravenous tacrolimus was started intraoperatively and continued for the first 2 days, and then changed to an oral dose. To maintain whole blood levels using microparticle enzyme immunoassay (MEIA) technology, around 20 ng/ml was given during the 1st month, 10–15 ng/ml during the following 5 months, and 5–10 ng/ml thereafter. 3. Azathioprine (Imuran) was initially given at a dose of 2 mg/kg/day, and the dose was then adapted to the blood neutrophil and/or lymphocyte count. Monoclonal antibodies directed against interleukin-2 receptors (anti-R-IL2 mAb) were administered to the last two small bowel recipients (Simulect, Novartis, Switzerland). All recipients were treated with intravenous antibiotics until intestinal transit recovery, and received total bowel decontamination for 1 month postoperatively and in cases of acute graft rejection. Antiinfective prophylaxis also included acyclovir or ganciclovir during the first three postoperative months. Quantitative Epstein-Barr virus (EBV) polymerase chain reaction (PCR) was performed weekly in the peripheral blood. Allograft biopsies were performed every other day from the 6th postoperative day to the end of the 3rd week, and according to clinical events thereafter. All biopsy specimens were examined histopathologically and immunohistochemically.

Oral and/or enteral feeding using a gastrostomy tube was started from the end of the first postoperative week using lactose and fiber-free diets with a low content of long-chain triglycerides. Standard parenteral nutrition formulas were tapered off gradually as oral or enteral feeding was advanced according to digestive tolerance and weight gain.

Results

The overall patient and primary graft survival rates at 6 months, and 1 and 3 years were 77% for patients, and 75%, 62%, and 59%, respectively, for grafts. Thirteen (40%) of the 32 grafts were lost either by recipient death ($n = 7$) or as a result of intestinal graft enterectomy ($n = 6$). For ITx, the actuarial patient and graft survival rates at 6 months, and 1 and 3 years were 75% for patients, and 67%, 42%, and 33%, respectively, for grafts. With LITx, four patients' grafts died within the first 2 months following transplantation, and one patient underwent retransplantation 4 months after primary transplantation. Thus, actuarial patient and graft survival rates at 6 months were 79% and 75%, respectively, and were the same at 1 and 3 years. Graft survival after LITx was significantly higher than after isolated ITx ($P < 0.02$). Right colon grafting did not affect patient or graft survival with either ITx or LITx transplantation. Neither clinical nor histological manifestations of graft-versus-host disease (GVHD) were observed. Rejection of the intestinal allograft occurred 17 times in 12 patients (8 LITx). The first episode of intestinal rejection appeared at a median of 15 days (range 3–22 days). All but four episodes of intestinal rejection were successfully treated by increasing tacrolimus dosages and giving a 3-day methylprednisolone bolus. Three patients received antilymphoglobulins (Pasteur–Mérieux, France) at a dosage of 5 mg/kg/day for 10 days. One (LITx) of these three patients died from sepsis, and two ITx recipients underwent graft removal. Acute liver rejection proved by liver biopsy occurred six times in six patients during the first 2 months, and was successfully treated using a 3-day methylprednisolone bolus. Because of abnormal liver function tests between 2 and 18 months following transplantation, six children underwent liver biopsy. These showed abnormal liver histological patterns suggestive of chronic liver rejection. These patients were treated using methylprednisolone and azathioprine or mycophenolate mofetil.

Surgical complications occurred in 20 recipients, and were more frequent in LITx than in ITx recipients (85% vs. 25%; $P < 0.05$). They included intestinal perforation, intestinal bleeding, biliary leak or stenosis, hepatic artery thrombosis, intraabdominal abscess, intestinal graft volvulus, eventration, and chylous ascites. The first three recipients presented with reversible EBV-associated posttransplant lymphoproliferative disease (PTLD). Two LITx recipients presented with lymphoma (mediastinal, intestinal) 3 and 18 months after transplantation. Both resolved by decreasing immunosuppression and using anti-CD-20 monoclonal antibodies. Cytomegalovirus (CMV) disease developed in six patients and was resolved by using protracted ganciclovir treatment.

Feeding was introduced at a median of 9 days posttransplant (range 6–62). Eighteen of 19 children (95%) had been weaned from parenteral nutrition

3–30 weeks after grafting. All total parenteral nutrition (TPN)-weaned recipients gained weight and have recovered normal growth velocity.

Discussion

Data from the Intestinal Transplantation Registry [7, 8] as well as from individual programs [9–16] show that the prognosis after intestinal transplantation has improved during the past 10 years. Interestingly, from our experience, the most encouraging results have been after LITx. Despite the severity of the illness, extent of operation performed, and higher incidence of surgical and infectious complications, 3-year patient and graft survivals after LITx were 79% and 75%, respectively. The mechanism by which the liver might reduce the risk of intestinal graft rejection is unknown. Isolated small bowel grafts not only have the highest incidence of rejection, but also require more intense immunosuppression to control it. From the registry as well as from the largest centers, it is currently difficult to analyze the difference in survival rates between isolated and combined liver ITx [9–15]. In general, the clinical status of liver–small bowel recipients is poor at the time of transplantation, and this contributes to the high posttransplant rate of morbidity and mortality [13]. This is suggested by the 1- and 2-year survival rates of patients who have not undergone transplantation being 30% and 22%, respectively, and the high number of deaths of patients on the waiting list [17–19]. Beath et al. [18] reported a marked discrepancy in clinical status between children referred for ITx from centers with and without nutritional care teams. In a recent study [19], the mortality rate, i.e., death within 6 months of evaluation for transplantation, was 90% in children with a short gut, 50% in those with mucosal disease, and 40% in those with chronic intestinal pseudoobstruction syndrome. Factors impacting on the survival of children with intestinal failure referred for ITx have been studied in patients evaluated for intestinal transplantation [17]. Only 82 (32%) underwent transplantation (68 liver-small bowel transplantation) with a mean waiting time of 10.1 ± 1.3 months. Of the 175 patients who were not transplanted, 120 died. The main factors associated with poor prognosis were age below 1 year, surgical disease, bridging fibrosis or cirrhosis, bilirubin levels of over 3 mg/dl, and thrombocytopenia. In our experience, the time taken to change from portal fibrosis to cirrhosis is approximately 12 months, which is similar to the transplantation waiting time [20]. Once cirrhosis has been established, survival at 1 year is only 30% [17]. It is well established that patients referred for liver-small bowel transplantation are more debilitated, have multiple complications, and have prolonged stays in the intensive care unit [21]. This may explain the lower patient and graft survival rates compared with those for isolated small bowel transplantation reported from several programs [13, 15].

Infectious complications after ITx are frequent and sometimes fatal. Rejection and sepsis can be intimately related after ITx when rejection compromises the normal intestinal barrier mechanisms and bacterial translocation results in consequent multiorgan failure [22]. Five recipients died from sepsis following treatment for acute rejection, including the use of antilymphoglobulins for steroid-resistant rejection in two cases. Viral infections such as CMV primoinfection or reactivation are frequent, and cannot always be prevented by the use of preemptive treatment. PCR is a sensitive method for the early detection of CMV infection in intestinal graft recipients [23]. The incidence of CMV infection, which was 19% in this series, has been reported to be as high as 29% of pediatric recipients of intestinal grafts [24]. CMV prophylaxis is now well established with the widespread use of ganciclovir [25]. EBV-induced PTLD was reported to be particularly frequent (15%) in a series of intestinal graft recipients [26]. In the case of lymphoma, the use of anti-CD20 monoclonal antibodies has proved to be efficient in reversing the disease in two patients who are still alive with functioning grafts. However, donor selection and the prevention of EBV infection remain unsolved problems [27, 28].

Full nutritional autonomy with complete discontinuation of PN may be achieved in the majority of survivors. The delay in achieving full nutritional autonomy was longer in this series than in others [13–15]. Whatever the type of procedure used, long-term graft absorptive function is dependent on the effects of denervation, lymphatic disruption, immunosuppressive treatment, rejection, and infection [29]. Feeding must resume as early as possible after transplantation, either by mouth or by an enteral tube if the patient refuses to eat. Very few studies have focused on intestinal graft function [30]. Normal growth represents the best evidence of normal graft function. Finally, when rejection is controlled and infection avoided, graft survival allows PN weaning and a return to almost normal life.

ITx might be considered for children with permanent intestinal failure for whom all attempts to improve intestinal adaptation have been unsucessful [1]. However, the first treatment for intestinal failure is PN, and many patients may be maintained sucessfully in this way by specialist units [3]. As PN is generally well tolerated, even for long periods, each indication for transplantation must be carefully weighed. Thus, patient selection requires precise criteria for diagnosing irreversible intestinal failure, and an appropriate referral time for assessment and transplantation.

References

1. Goulet O (1998) Intestinal failure in children. Transplant Proc 30:2523–2525
2. Ricour C, Gorski AM, Goulet O, et al. (1990) Home parenteral nutrition in children: 8 years of experience with 112 patients. Clin Nutr 9:65–71

3. Colomb V, Goulet O, Ricour C (1998) Home enteral and parenteral nutrition. Baillière's Clin Gastroenterol 122:877–894

4. Goulet O, Michel JL, Jan D, et al. (1997) Intestinal transplantation in pediatric patients: the European experience. Transplant Proc 29:1785–1786

5. Goulet O, Révillon Y, Brousse N, et al. (1992) Successful small bowel transplantation in an infant. Transplantation 53:940–943

6. Todo S, Tsakis A, Abu-Elmagd K, et al. (1992) Cadaveric small bowel and small bowel–liver transplantation in humans. Transplantation 53:369–376

7. Grant D (1996) Intestinal Transplantation Registry on behalf of the current results of intestinal transplantation. Lancet 347:1801–1803

8. Grant D (1999) Intestinal transplantation: 1997 report of the International Registry. Transplantation 15:1061–1064

9. Langnas AN, Shaw BW, Antonson DL, et al. (1996) Preliminary experience with intestinal transplantation in infants and children. Pediatrics 97:443–448

10. Karatzas T, Khan F, Tzakis AG (1997) Clinical intestinal transplantation—experience in Miami. Transplant Proc 29:1787–1789

11. Atkison P, Williams S, Wall S, et al. (1998) Results of pediatric small bowel transplantation in Canada. Transplant Proc 30:2521–2522

12. Abu-Elmagd K, Reyes J, Todo S, et al. (1998) Clinical intestinal transplantation: new perspectives and immunologic considerations. J Am Coll Surg 186:512–525

13. Reyes J, Bueno J, Kocoshis S, et al. (1998) Current status of intestinal transplantation in children. J Pediatr Surg 243–254

14. Farmer DG, McDiarmid SV, Smith C, et al. (1998) Experience with combined liver–small intestine transplantation at the University of California, Los Angeles. Transplant Proc 30:2533–2534

15. Sudan DL, Kaufman S, Shaw BW, et al. (2000) Intestinal transplantation: for intestinal failure. Am J Gastroenterol 95:1506–1515

16. Goulet O, Jan D, Lacaille F, et al. (1999) Intestinal transplantation in children: preliminary experience in Paris. J Parenter Enter Nutr 23(Suppl.):S121–S125

17. Bueno J, Ohwada S, Kocoshis S, et al. (1999) Factors impacting the survival of children with intestinal failure referred for intestinal transplantation. J Pediatr Surg 34:27–33

18. Beath SV, Booth IW, Murphy MS, et al. (1995) Nutritional care and candidates for small bowel transplantation. Arch Dis Child 73:348–350

19. Beath SV, Brook GA, Kelly DA, et al. (1998) Demand for pediatric small bowel transplantation in the United Kingdom. Transplant Proc 30:2531–2532

20. Colomb V, Jobert A, Lacaille F, et al. (1999) Parenteral nutrition associated liver disease in children: natural history and prognosis. J Pediatr Gastroenterol Nutr 28:577 (abstract)

21. Filston HC, Colombani PM (1996) Preliminary experience with intestinal transplantation in infants and children. Pediatrics 97:583–584

22. Goulet O, Brousse N, Révillon Y, et al. (1993) Pathology of human intestinal transplantation. In: Grant D, Wood RFM (eds) Small bowel transplantation. Edward Arnold, London, pp 112–120

23. Kusne S, Manez R, Frye BL, et al. (1997) Use of DNA amplification for diagnosis of cytomegalovirus enteritis after intestinal transplantation. Gastroenterology 112:1121–1128

24. Green M, Bueno J, Sigurdsson L, et al. (1999) Unique aspects of the infectious complications of intestinal transplantation. Curr Opin Organ Transplant 4:361–367

25. Patel R, Snydman DR, Rubin RH, et al. (1996) Cytomegalovirus prophylaxis in solid organ transplant recipients. Transplantation 61:1279–1289

26. Reyes J, Tzakis A, Bonet H, et al. (1994) Lymphoproliferative disease after intestinal transplantation under primary FK 506 immunosuppression. Transplant Proc 26: 1426–1427
27. Finn L, Reyes J, Bueno J, et al. (1998) Epstein–Barr virus infection in children after transplantation of the small intestine. Am J Surg Pathol 22:299–309
28. Green M, Reyes J, Jabbour N, et al. (1996) Use of quantitative PCR to predict onset of Epstein–Barr viral infection and post-transplant lymphoproliferative disease after intestinal transplantation in children. Transplant Proc 28:2759–2760
29. Kim J, Fryer J, Craig RM (1998) Absorptive function following small intestinal transplantation. Dig Dis Sci 43:1925–1930
30. Kaufman SS, Lyden ER, Brown CR, et al. (2000) Disaccharidase activities and fat assimilation in pediatric patients after intestinal transplantation. Transplantation 15:362–365

Living-Donor Small Bowel Transplantation: Experience of Three Cases

S. Uemoto[1], S. Kaihara[1], A. Yokoi[2], H. Oike[2], M. Kasahara[1], and K. Tanaka[1,2]

Summary. A living-donor small bowel transplantation (SBT) was performed in three cases with short-bowel syndrome. In all cases, the donor was the patient's mother and blood type combinations were identical. The distal 100 cm, 120 cm, and 140 cm of the ileum were resected for the grafts. The donors were discharged from the hospital on postoperative days 15, 16, and 14, respectively. All had mild tenesmus, which resolved 6 months after the operation, but have had no nutritional problems. The three recipients were a boy aged 2 years and 6 months, a girl aged 4 years and 5 months, and a boy aged 3 years and 5 months.

Immunosuppression consisted of tacrolimus, steroids, and azathioprine or cyclophosphamide. Induction treatment with a 3-day course of OKT3 or a 6-month course of daclizumab was given to the second and third case, respectively. The first patient experienced four episodes of rejection, and died of *Pneumocystis carinii* pneumonia 16 months after transplantation. The autopsy findings showed chronic rejection of the intestinal graft. The second recipient left the hospital completely weaned from total parenteral nutrition (TPN), but she later was readmitted with severe rejection. The graft had developed chronic rejection and was removed. This patient received a cadaveric SBT 8 months after removal of the living-donor graft. The third recipient had one episode of mild rejection, which was easily treated with a steroid bolus. He was discharged from hospital completely weaned from TPN 5 months after transplantation.

In our experience, harvesting of the distal ileum as an intestinal graft can be performed safely. Rejection is still the main obstacle to a successful outcome.

Key words. Small bowel transplantation, Living donor

---

[1]Organ Transplant Unit, and [2]Department of Transplantation and Immunology, Kyoto University Hospital, 54 Kawahara-cho, Shogoin, Sakyo-ku, Kyoto 606-8507, Japan

Small bowel transplantation (SBT) has become a realistic treatment for patients with intestinal failure since the introduction of tacrolimus [1] and anti-CD25 antibody (daclizumab) [2]. A living-donor SBT was performed in three cases with short-bowel syndrome. The second case also received a cadaveric SBT following a failed living-donor SBT.

Donors

In all cases, the donor was the patient's mother (case 1, 31 years old; case 2, 32 years old; case 3, 28 years old), the blood type combination was identical, and human leukocyte antigen combinations were haploidentical. The distal ileum (100 cm, 120 cm, and 140 cm, respectively) was harvested, and the ileocolic vessels and the ileocecal valve were left intact. The grafts were perfused with cold University of Wisconsin (UW) solution. One donor experienced intestinal obstruction on the 5th postoperative day, which resolved spontaneously on the 8th postoperative day. The donors were discharged from the hospital on postoperative days 15, 16, and 14, respectively. All donors had mild tenesmus, which resolved 6 months after the operation, but have had no nutritional problems.

Recipient 1

A boy who was 2 years and 6 months old and who had short-bowel syndrome underwent SBT due to the loss of central venous access. The graft vessels were anastomosed to the recipient's aorta and infrarenal inferior vena cava (IVC) in an end-to-side fashion. Immunosuppression consisted of tacrolimus, steroids, and azathioprine. The patient experienced four episodes of rejection, and was on total parenteral nutrition (TPN) almost throughout his post-transplant course. He died of *Pneumocystis carinii* pneumonia 16 months after transplantation. The autopsy findings showed chronic rejection of the intestinal graft.

Recipient 2

A girl who was 4 years and 5 months old and who had short-bowel syndrome underwent SBT because of recurrent line sepsis and TPN-induced liver failure. Her pretransplant total bilirubin level was 8.0 mg/dl, and a liver biopsy showed severe fibrosis. The graft artery was anastomosed to the recipient's aorta and the vein to the inferior mesenteric vein because the recipient's infrarenal IVC was obliterated. Immunosuppression consisted of tacrolimus, steroids, and cyclophosphamide, with a 3-day course of OKT3 induction therapy. Her bilirubin level became normal within 10 days after transplantation. The patient experienced one episode of rejection, but left the hospital completely weaned from TPN 4 months after transplantation. Unfortunately, she was readmitted 1 month later with severe rejection. This rejection episode was controlled, but later she had two more rejection episodes that could not be resolved completely. The graft developed chronic rejection and was removed 21 months after transplantation. This patient received a cadaveric SBT 8 months after removal of the living-donor graft. This was the first case of cadaveric SBT in Japan. The donor was a 54-year-old woman, and the length of the graft was 240 cm. The graft was preserved in UW solution, and the cold ischemic time was 7 h 39 min. The graft vessels were anastomosed to the recipient's aorta and portal vein, respectively. Anti-CD25 antibody (daclizumab) was used as an induction treatment for 6 months. The patient was weaned from TPN 2 months after the cadaveric SBT. She experienced a moderate degree of rejection and cytomregalovirus enteritis 4 and 5 months after transplantation, respectively. Both episodes were completely resolved, and she is now awaiting discharge from the hospital.

Recipient 3

A boy who was 3 years and 5 months old, and who had short-bowel syndrome, underwent living-donor SBT due to loss of venous access. The graft vein was anastomosed to the recipient's splenic vein because of the obliteration of the recipient's infrarenal IVC. Triple immunosuppression (tacrolimus, steroids, and cyclophosphamide) with a 6-month course of daclizumab was instituted. The patient had one episode of mild rejection, which was easily treated with a steroid bolus. He was discharged from the hospital completely weaned from TPN 5 months after the transplantation. The patient is now thriving on a normal diet with a functioning graft.

Conclusions

From our experience, harvesting of the distal ileum as an intestinal graft can be performed safely. Rejection is still the main obstacle to a successful outcome, but immunosuppression with daclizumab may overcome the failures of other drugs.

References

1. Todo S, Reyes J, Furukawa H, et al. (1995) Outcome analysis of 71 clinical intestinal transplantations. Ann Surg 222:270–282
2. Abu-Elmagd K, Fung J, McGhee W, et al. (2000) The efficacy of daclizumab for intestinal transplantation: preliminary report. Transplant Proc 32:1195–1196

Small Bowel Transplantation as a Final Treatment for Intestinal Failure

Akira Okada, Toshimichi Hasegawa, Masafumi Wasa, and Tatsuo Azuma

Summary. As a consequence of recent advances in long-term total parenteral nutrition (TPN), intestinal failure has come to be recognized as an established pathological entity. However, a number of problems remain to be answered before long-term TPN is widely and safely performed. The most serious and important of these are catheter-related sepsis and liver dysfunction. When it becomes impossible to continue TPN because of these complications, small bowel transplantation (SBT) is considered as the treatment of choice. In Japan, the first SBT was performed in Kyoto in 1998, and since then three more cases, including this one, have followed. The case we treated is that of a 16-year-old boy with a diagnosis of microvillus inclusion disease who had been receiving long-term TPN for persistent diarrhea since birth. When he developed liver dysfunction with hepatosplenomegaly, a living-related intestinal transplantation was performed, with the donor being his 59-year-old blood-matched grandmother. The postoperative course was uneventful. Enteral feeding was started on postoperative day 14, and later he was switched to an oral diet. TPN was discontinued 5 months postoperatively, and he is doing well so far.

Regarding the number of candidates for intestinal transplantation in Japan, an annual survey of patients receiving home parenteral nutrition is available from the Registry Promotion Committee of the Japanese Society for Home Parenteral Nutrition (HPN). According to the latest survey in 2000, a total of 355 patients (malignant, 202; benign, 149) are presently receiving HPN. If we assume that half of the patients with benign disease would potentially be real candidates for SBT, there would be 75 patients on the list.

Department of Pediatric Surgery, Osaka University Graduate School of Medicine, 2-2 Yamadaoka, Suita, Osaka 565-0871, Japan

Key words. Small bowel transplantation, Total parenteral nutrition, Intestinal failure, Short bowel syndrome, Home parenteral nutrition

Recent advances in total parenteral nutrition (TPN) have made it possible to rehabilitate patients with an extensive loss of intestinal function. Consequently, the concept of "intestinal failure," defined as a reduction of the functioning gut mass, has come to be recognized as an established pathological entity [1, 2]. The records show that TPN was first performed in our University Hospital in 1971. We have now established a well-coordinated team of TPN personnel such as physicians, nurses, pharmacists, and dietitians, who regularly visit all in-patients receiving TPN, can be consulted in cases of difficulty or emergency, and hold regular nutrition conferences [3]. This system led to a rapid recognition throughout the whole hospital of the need for nutritional support. Many more patients are now receiving TPN, as shown in Fig. 1. To date, about 5000 patients have been treated under this system.

The clinical indications for TPN and the numbers of patients affected are summarized in Table 1. As can be seen, perioperative management, including postoperative complications, accounted for over 40% of the patients, and anticancer treatment accounted for a further 25%. One unusual indication is "intestinal failure," the existence of which came to be recognized as TPN became more widely used. In Japan, intravenous infusion was not officially allowed except in hospital until 1985, when the Ministry of Health and Welfare

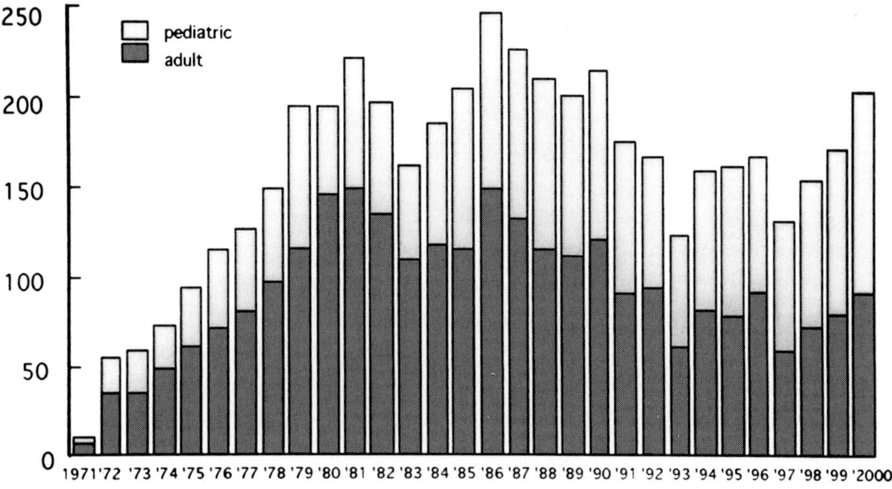

FIG. 1. Number of cases of total parenteral nutrition in 30 years of experience. Osaka University Hospital, March 2001

TABLE 1. Clinical indications for total parenteral nutrition (1971–2000, Osaka University Hospital)

	Adult	Pediatric	Total
Perioperative management	811	1004	1815 (36.4%)
Postoperative complications	209	83	292 (5.9%)
GI symptoms (ileus, diarrhea, bleeding)	232	163	395 (7.9%)
Inadequate oral intake	457	100	557 (11.2%)
Anticancer therapy	742	515	1257 (25.2%)
Hepatic or renal failure	101	29	130 (2.6%)
Respiratory failure	96	77	173 (3.5%)
Intestinal failure	90	91	181 (3.6%)
Others	134	52	186 (3.7%)
Total	2872	2114	4986

GI, gastrointestinal

TABLE 2. Indications for long-term parenteral nutrition in intestinal failure (70 cases) (March 2001, Osaka University Hospital)

Adult ($n = 30$)		Pediatric ($n = 40$)	
Short bowel syndrome	12	Short bowel syndrome	13
		Massive intestinal resection	8
		Extensive aganglionosis	5
Bowel dysfunctions	18	Bowel dysfunctions	27
Crohn's disease	9	Infantile diarrheal diseases	21
CIIPS[a]	6	Hypoganglionosis	2
Nonspecific intestinal ulcers	2	Motor disorders	2
Behçet's disease	1	Crohn's disease	1
		CIIPS[a]	1

[a] Chronic idiopathic intestinal pseudoobstruction syndrome

approved the use of home parenteral nutrition and agreed that it should be covered by the medical insurance system [4]. As a result, such patients became socially rehabilitated and enjoyed their daily life again. The number of patients who could return home from medical centers all over Japan then increased rapidly.

Excluding cases who received TPN only once, a total of 70 patients, 30 adult and 40 pediatric, have received prolonged TPN for intestinal failure in our department during the past 30 years. Intestinal failure can roughly be classified into two categories: short bowel syndrome; and bowel dysfunction. Table 2 shows the indications for the patients in each category where long-term TPN was performed for intestinal failure. Of the 30 adult patients, 12 (39%) had short bowel syndrome, mostly due to ischemic disease of the intestine. The other 18 patients had bowel dysfunctions such as Crohn's disease (9 cases), chronic pseudoobstruction (6 cases), nonspecific multiple intestinal ulcers (2 cases), or Behçet's disease (1 case). Of the 40 pediatric patients, 13 (32.5%) had short bowel syndrome, mostly due to congenital anomalies such as jejunoileal atresia, or mid-gut volvulus. The other 27 patients had infantile diarrhea (21 cases), hypoganglionosis (2 cases), motor disorders (2 cases), Crohn's disease (1 case), or chronic idiopathic intestinal pseudoobstruction syndrome (1 case). The total period of TPN varied, but in 13 cases it extended over 10 years, and the longest was 26 years.

Of the 70 cases described above, 25 patients (35.7%) were weaned from TPN, 28 patients (40%) were still on TPN, and 16 patients died during treatment. The remaining patient recently received a small bowel transplantation (SBT). There is a significant difference in clinical outcome between pediatric and adult patients. In pediatric patients, 55% were weaned off TPN, whereas in adult patients, only 10% were weaned off TPN (Fig. 2). Among patients with short bowel syndrome, no adult patients were weaned off TPN, whereas 7 of 13 (54%) pediatric patients were weaned off TPN (Fig. 3). This could be due

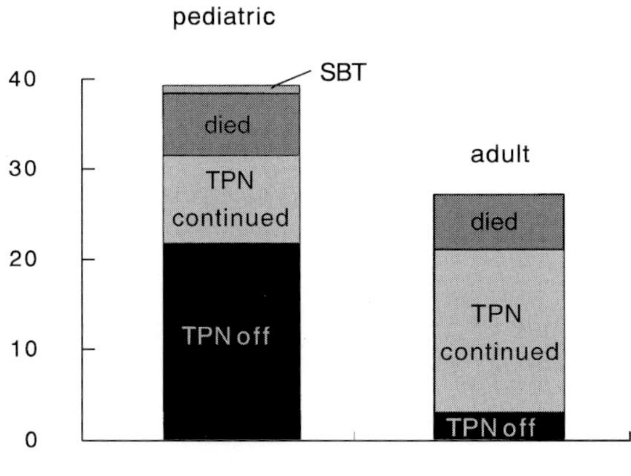

FIG. 2. Outcome of intestinal failure in 70 patients (1971–2000, Department of Pediatric Surgery, Osaka University Hospital)

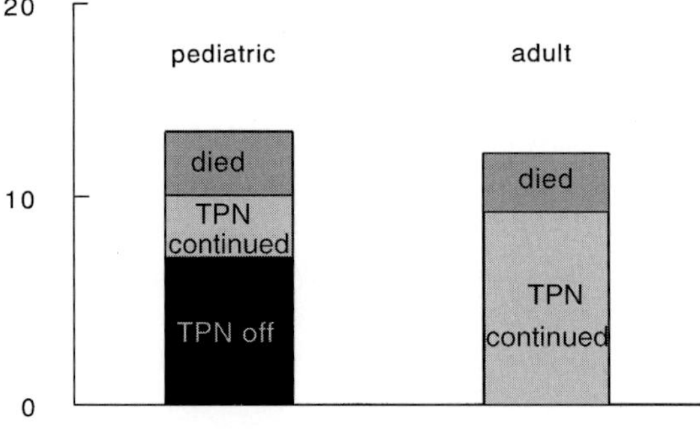

FIG. 3. Outcome of intestinal failure (short bowel syndrome) in 25 patients (1971–2000, Department of Pediatric Surgery, Osaka University Hospital)

to a remarkable capacity for mucosal adaptation during childhood [5, 6]. Of the 16 patients who died during treatment, the most frequent cause of death was central venous catheter-related sepsis in 8 and irreversible hepatic failure in 3. The remaining 5 patients probably died from their original disease.

The case of SBT is described here. A 16-year-old boy had experienced severe diarrhea since birth, and had never responded to any type of treatment. Consequently, he was nourished by TPN at home. A biopsy specimen from his intestine showed microvillus inclusion bodies. Because of meticulous daily management of the catheter and metabolic care by the team, as well as total cooperation by his family, he enjoyed a high-quality social life. However, at 14 years of age, he developed hepatosplenomegaly and abnormal liver function test. There was a marked decrease in prothrombin time. The peripheral blood platelet count was $39 \times 10^3/mm^3$. A liver biopsy specimen showed marked fatty infiltration with bridging fibrosis. Because of the progressive deterioration of liver function, his condition was judged to indicate SBT. The patient's 59-year-old, blood-type-matched grandmother offered to be a living related donor. The SBT was performed on March 27, 2000. A 150-cm-long ileal graft was harvested from the donor, the small bowel of the recipient from Treitz's ligament to the terminal ileum was resected, and the graft was interposed with vascular reconstruction. Immunosuppression with combined tacrolimus, daclizumab, cyclophosphamide, and a low-dose steroid was carried out. Just over 1 year later, the patient's condition is reasonably good and he can now tolerate regular oral meals.

The annual survey of patients receiving home parenteral nutrition by the Registry Promotion Committee of the Japanese Society for Home Parenteral Nutrition (HPN) gives the actual number of candidates for intestinal transplantation in Japan [7]. According to the latest survey taken in 2000, a total of 355 patients (malignant, 202; benign, 149) are presently receiving HPN. Table 3 shows the number of patients with benign diseases classified according to the categories for which long-term TPN is required. It can be assumed that about half these patients (70–80 cases) might be candidates for SBT. As mentioned above, there are some patients with intestinal failure for whom TPN is the only way to sustain life. Since this situation is often complicated by recurrent infections of the central venous line, loss of venous access, and irreversible hepatic fibrosis, intestinal transplantation becomes the only life-saving alternative. Although previous clinical results have been discouraging despite its technical feasibility, the recent development of new immunosuppressants has produced a significant improvement in graft survival [8]. Last year, the Japanese government reconsidered its importance as an organ transplant, and added "intestine" to the organ procurement program, which already included kidney, liver, heart, lung, and pancreas. Table 4 shows the criteria for the selection of recipients according to the emergency

TABLE 3. Japanese survey of home parenteral nutrition in 1999 (Japanese Society for Home Parenteral Nutrition, recorded in 2000)

Benign diseases	149 (61)
Inflammatory bowel disease	36 (12)
Crohn's disease	31 (9)
Ulcerative colitis	3 (2)
Nonspecific multiple intestinal ulcers	2 (1)
Ischemic diseases	38 (36)
SMA embolism	12 (12)
Volvulus	17 (16)
Strangulation ileus	9 (8)
Motor disorders	34 (10)
CIIPS	12 (2)
MMIHS	1
Neuronal intestinal dysplasia	1
Hirschsprung and allied disease	18 (7)
Others	2 (1)
Other GI diseases	19 (3)
Intractable diarrhea	5
Others	14 (3)
Others	22

SMA, superior mesenteric artery
Figures for short bowel syndrome are shown in parentheses

TABLE 4. Criteria for the selection of recipients for small bowel transplantation (September 2000, Ministry of Health and Welfare)

1. The ranking of medical emergency
   Status 1: inability to maintain central venous route
   Status 2: hyperbilirubinemic with progressive liver
             failure
   Status 3: exhausted central venous route

2. ABO blood type

3. Waiting time

ranking established by a committee organized by the Ministry of Health, Labor and Welfare.

In Japan, clinical intestinal transplantation has been performed in 5 cases to date (4 patients: 3 in Kyoto and 1 in Osaka). Two developed severe rejection of the graft, which was removed postoperatively, and one of these later died. The remaining cases are doing well so far. These results are promising now that new immunosuppressive agents, as well as tacrolimus, are available, and meticulous postoperative management, with direct observation of graft mucosa by zoom-endoscopy, is possible.

In Japan, after three decades of struggle, transplantation of the small intestine is finally emerging as a viable clinical option. We have already established a very safe TPN maintenance system. We hope that in the near future SBT will become an established treatment for intestinal failure as an alternative to TPN.

References

1. Irving M (1956) Ethical problems associated with the treatment of intestinal failure. Aust NZ Surg 56:425–427
2. Okada A, Takagi Y, Fukuzawa M, Nezu R (1994) Intestinal failure–its nature, pathophysiology and treatment. Asia Pacific J Clin Nutr 3:3–8.
3. Okada A (1982) Total parenteral nutrition in gastroenterological surgery: its appropriate indication and limitation. Asian Med J 25:199–226
4. Takagi Y, Okada A, Sato T, et al. (1995) A report on the first annual survey of home parenteral nutrition in Japan. Surg Today 25:193–201
5. Wilmore DW, Dudrick SJ, Daly JM, Vars HM (1971) The role of nutrition in the adaptation of the small intestine after massive small bowel resection. Surg Gynecol Obstet 132:673–680
6. Dowling RH (1982) Small bowel adaptation and its regulation. Scand J Gastroenterol 17:53–73
7. Registry Promotion Committee of the Japanese Society for Home Parenteral Nutrition (2000) Annual survey of home parenteral nutrition in Japan
8. Proceedings of the Fifth International Symposium on Small Bowel Transplantation (1998) Transplant Proc 30:2509–2685

Part 4
Liver Transplantation for Malignant Hepatic Tumors

The Role of Liver Transplantation in the Treatment of Primary Liver Tumors

PETER NEUHAUS and SVEN JONAS

Summary. From a worldwide perspective, hepatocellular carcinoma (HCC) and cholangiocarcinoma account for 84% and 13% of all primary liver tumors, respectively. Liver transplantation has resulted in poor results when used for non-cirrhotic patients suffering from either HCC or cholangiocarcinoma. The only exception is fibrolamellar carcinoma; whether this is an indication for liver transplantation is still under consideration. The tumor indication with the most favorable survival rate is early HCC in cirrhosis. Vascular invasion is the most serious risk factor, but its detection is still impossible prior to the histopathological examination of a specimen. Therefore, surrogate markers are required. Stringent selection criteria relating to size and number of tumor nodules have been identified and must be adhered to in order to avoid recurrence. Recurrence is especially harmful in the transplant population because the immunosuppressive treatment appears to reduce the time taken for the tumor to double in volume.

Another major problem for liver transplantation as a therapy for malignancy is an increasing shortage of donor grafts. This situation may be changed by a wider introduction of living-donor liver transplantation among adults. To date, there are no reports on the outcome after adult living-donor liver transplantations for extended, or even critical, indications of HCC.

Key words. Liver transplantation, Hepatocellular carcinoma, Fibrolamellar carcinoma, Cholangiocarcinoma, Cirrhosis

Department of General, Visceral and Transplantation Surgery, Charité, Campus Virchow Clinic, Humboldt University, Augustenburger Platz 1, 13353 Berlin, Germany

Introduction

Hepatocellular carcinoma (HCC) is by far the most prevalent primary liver tumor, with the next most prevalent being cholangiocarcinoma. Other primary hepatic neoplasms are rarely encountered in surgical practice. From a worldwide perspective, HCC and cholangiocarcinoma account for 84% and 13% of all primary liver tumors, respectively [1]. To date, surgical resection has been the main treatment for primary liver tumors, as it may provide consistent long-term tumor-free survival. Postoperative mortality, as well as fatalities due to a recurrence of the tumor and complications from cirrhosis, have impaired outcomes, especially in the treatment of HCC in cirrhosis. Other therapeutic practices, such as total hepatectomy and liver transplantation, percutaneous ethanol injection, transarterial chemoembolization, laser-induced thermotherapy, radiofrequency thermoablation, and photodynamic therapy have also resulted in favorable survival figures, at least in part, and could emphasize the need for a revision of standardized therapeutic strategies [2–6].

Almost all of these investigations have aimed at an improvement in the therapy for HCC, whereas cholangiocarcinoma has only rarely been a focus of interest. This neglect is only partially due to its relative rarity when compared with HCC. It is also relevant that cholangiocarcinoma is linked to chronic liver diseases to a much lesser extent than HCC, and therefore is only detected by chance as a small subclinical and resectable mass.

Liver Transplantation

One major problem for liver transplantation as a therapy for malignancy is an increasing shortage of donor grafts. If the outcome after liver transplantation for primary HCC is considered not in terms of posttransplant survival, but by an intention-to-treat analysis of all patients with HCC on the transplant waiting list, the favorable survival figures become considerably lower because of drop-outs during the extended waiting time [7]. The reason for this is that tumors progress with a 1-year-probability of 70%. The 1-year-rates for vascular invasion and extrahepatic spread are 21% and 9%, respectively [8].

This situation may be changed by a wider use of living-donor liver transplantation among adults. The most important difference from cadaveric transplantation is that each graft is uniquely available for one recipient. An allocation according to the most favorable outcome, which would generally be anticipated for benign liver diseases rather than HCC, is not only not necessary, but is impossible. In Germany at least, existing legislation covers living-donor organ transplantation only between closely related persons. The prognosis for a patient with HCC which is too advanced according to the selection criteria described above, can not be compared with the expected outcome of other potential graft recipients but only with the prognosis provided by other therapeutic options. There are no reports on outcomes after adult living-donor liver transplantation for extended, or even critical, indications related to HCC. Nevertheless, it can be expected that transplantation in cases of recurrent HCC in cirrhosis after resection would be indicated less stringently. The most important caveat is the risk of complications for the donor, who is not a patient but a healthy individual.

Hepatocellular Carcinoma in Cirrhosis

Only half of the patients dying in the course of this disease do so due to the liver tumor or its metastases. The other patients die from the underlying chronic liver disease [9]. Liver transplantation is the only simultaneous treatment for primary liver disease as well as HCC. As about 80% of all HCCs develop within cirrhotic liver tissue, which is considered to be a risk factor for malignant transformation, most patients have to be evaluated regarding the therapeutic potential of liver transplantation with respect to their primary disease. The problem of de novo HCC within cirrhotic livers, or of small satellites which have been overlooked, has been addressed by Belghiti et al. [10]. An analysis of 47 patients after liver resection of HCC and cirrhosis, with a clear resection margin of at least 1 cm, showed an intrahepatic recurrence rate of 60% ($n = 28$). Most (86%) recurrent intrahepatic tumors were detected within a distance to the resection margin of at least 2 cm. The overall 5-year survival after liver resection was 17%.

A crucial factor requiring further investigation is the appropriate selection of patients. The tumor-node-metastasis (TNM) and Union Internationale Contre le Cancer (UICC) classifications of HCC must be considered with caution for therapeutic decision making because they refer to biologically different tumors in common categories, e.g., carcinomas with and without vascular invasion in T stages 2–4. Selection should not allow patients in whom the cancer has extended beyond hepatic confines to become candidates for liver transplantation. Gross metastases or lymph node infiltration, which are indicators of extrahepatic spread, are easily detectable by pretransplant imaging procedures or laparoscopic staging [11, 12]. However, the current state of pretransplant and even intraoperative diagnostic imaging still fails to distinguish reliably between patients with HCC in cirrhosis with or without vascular infiltration. In liver transplantation, the problem of microscopic tumor cell dissemination is of great importance because posttransplantation immunosuppression appears to alter tumor cell kinetics. The increased risk of intrahepatic recurrence and limited survival under immunosuppression has been shown in a study by Yokoyama et al. [13], who found a much shorter tumor volume doubling time (TVDT) in recurrent HCCs after transplantation than after resection (33 ± 7 vs. 274 ± 79 days).

Bismuth et al. [14] were the first to show that in the earliest liver transplantations, the surgical strategy for the treatment of HCC in cirrhosis had followed a misconception in selecting patients with advanced, and therefore unresectable, cancers as transplant candidates. Even groups advocating the continuation of liver transplantation as a therapeutic option for selected patients with unresectable liver tumors of various anatomic origins recommended excluding UICC Stages III and IV HCCs from liver transplantation alone [15]. Based on the United Network of Organ Sharing (UNOS) and the European Liver Transplant Registry (ELTR) data, it can be seen that patient survival was poor, and reached only 30% 5 years posttransplant. Conversely, small HCCs in cirrhosis, with diameters of less than 3 cm and comprising only one or two nodules, i.e., tumors normally suitable for resection, showed favorable outcomes.

The most favorable results originate from groups applying selection criteria that do not adhere stringently to the TNM classification, but instead consider the size and number of tumor nodules. Patients with HCC and cirrhosis with three tumor nodules or fewer, a maximum diameter not exceeding 5 cm, and no signs of vascular invasion underwent the same evaluation process as is required for transplant candidates with other, mostly benign, indications for liver transplantation. Table 1 shows recently obtained survival data of groups from Milan and Barcelona as well as our own results [16–18]. These independently performed studies showed consistent 5-year survival rates

TABLE 1. Selection criteria and survival data from the centers in Milan, Barcelona, and Berlin

	Ref.	Selection criteria	n	5-year survival
Milan	16	Solitary tumors < 5 cm, 1–3 nodes < 3 cm	48	75%[a]
Barcelona	17	Solitary tumors < 5 cm, no vascular invasion	58	74%
Berlin	18	Solitary tumors < 5 cm, 1–3 nodes < 3 cm, no vascular invasion	120	70%

[a] 4-year survival

of more than 70%, and are likely to support these criteria as a marker for the absence of vascular infiltration.

In our experience, three factors account for this favorable long-term prognosis.

1. No operative fatalities occurred, whereas postoperative mortality ranges from 3% to 15% after liver resections performed in patients with cirrhosis.
2. The rates of tumor recurrence were low, and total hepatectomy is always considered to be formally curative. In particular, atypical or wedge resections performed because of limited functional hepatic reserves frequently do not succeed in achieving sufficiently clear resection margins, and bear the risk that satellite nodules may be overlooked. Moreover, total hepatectomy offers the chance of complete histopathological staging for the detection of multicentricity or small satellite nodules. In contrast, staging based on diagnostic imaging will probably generate false-negative results by missing some smaller satellites in the future remnant liver. Interestingly, the study by Bismuth et al. [14] also showed that the 3-year survival rate after resection of patients with small HCCs (<3 cm) in cirrhosis was only 39%, and was worse than the 3-year survival rate of 55% in those with larger nodules (>5 cm). The authors explained this puzzling paradox as an increased likelihood of undetected nodules in remnant liver tissue when only one or two small nodules were discovered by repeated screening. In experience of transplantation cases, the rate of pretransplant, undetected carcinomatous foci in cirrhotic livers was 24%. This figure has been confirmed by Mazzaferro et al. as well as by our own results [9, 16].
3. The fatal potential of underlying liver disease which may be deleterious after resection can almost be ignored after transplantation, except for a few patients with recurrent hepatitis B.

Other markers, more directly correlated to vascular infiltration, are needed to identify patients who, even though conforming to the selection criteria currently applied, do not benefit over the long term as well as those who are currently excluded owing to excessive strictness. Another possible strategy to assess the suitability of a patient may be pretransplantation transarterial chemoembolization (TACE). This is a concept which was more or less accidentally generated from a study on multimodal therapy. Bismuth and co-workers [19] conducted a retrospective analysis of their experience with TACE and failed to show any survival benefit. Interestingly, however, they demonstrated significant survival benefits by dividing the patients who were treated with TACE into one group that had responded with tumor necrosis, and one which had not developed necrosis. Therefore, it is worth investigating whether chemoembolization might serve as a selection criterion prior to liver transplantation.

It is still a matter of debate whether multimodal therapy will be able to improve outcomes [20]. To date, treatment options in conjunction with liver transplantation have been confined to pilot trials involving TACE and postoperative chemotherapy. Olthoff et al. [20] reported that doxorubicin pre-, intra-, and postoperatively showed a significant increase in survival rates when compared with historic controls. However, the tumor stages were not well defined, and 3-year survival rates did not compare favorably with those reported from many series without adjuvant therapy. Prospective randomized trials have not been published to date, although they are in progress at different centers.

Hepatocellular Carcinoma in Noncirrhotic Livers

In general, HCC in noncirrhotic livers occurs considerably less frequently than in cirrhosis, but these few tumors are much more advanced. In an autopsy study from Japan involving 618 patients, Okuda et al. [21] reported a rate of only 11% of HCC growing in non-cirrhotic livers. Few data are available on hepatocellular carcinomas in noncirrhotic livers because this type of tumor is rarely separately identified in series reported in the literature. One of the characteristics of this tumor is its advanced size at diagnosis.

In the largest single-center studies of the treatment of HCC in noncirrhotic livers, Bismuth et al. [22], in Paris, and Iwatsuki et al. [23], in Pittsburgh, reported 5-year survival rates after liver resection of 40% and 44%, respectively. We have reported a rate of 38% in patients with tumors in UICC stage III, which represent by far the largest group of patients still eligible for treatment with a curative intention [9]. However, some UICC IVa tumors may also undergo surgical therapy because the functional capacity of liver tissue frequently allows extended liver resections.

Attempts to improve the treatment of HCC in noncirrhotics by performing total hepatectomy and liver transplantation have failed. These advanced tumors are highly likely to disseminate microscopically, and in consequence have an overwhelming risk of recurrence, which is further increased by immunosuppression. The average rate of posttransplant 5-year survival is 26%, as reported by Pichlmayr et al. and Iwatsuki et al. [15, 23].

Fibrolamellar Carcinoma

In patients with fibrolamellar carcinoma, the recommendation not to perform liver transplantation in noncirrhotics needs to be further substantiated. Fibrolamellar carcinoma is an uncommon variant of HCC which is only exceptionally associated with cirrhosis, and is distinguished by histopathological features suggesting greater differentiation than other HCCs [24–26].

As most fibrolamellar carcinoma patients are young noncirrhotics, it is uncertain whether a better prognosis after liver resection when compared with that of patients with conventional HCC can be ascribed to the properties of the tumor. Data reported in the literature to date, which are from fewer than 200 patients assessed after surgical therapy, do not show conclusive results.

The largest single-center report originates from Pittsburgh. Pinna et al. [27] described the treatment of fibrolamellar carcinoma with resection ($n = 28$) or transplantation ($n = 13$) in 41 patients. The mean age of the patients was 30 years. Almost all fibrolamellar carcinomas could be assigned to UICC stages IVa or even IVb, with surprising postoperative 5-year survival rates of 66% and 50%, respectively. Comparing patients undergoing liver resection with those in whom liver transplantation had been performed, the 5-year survival rates were 82% and 38%, respectively. Liver resection was consistently superior to liver transplantation over the years, and the gap of 44% at 5 years also prevailed after 10 years. In our opinion, these outstanding results after the resection of advanced-stage fibrolamellar carcinoma may in fact indicate a prognosis which is different from that of nonfibrolamellar HCCs without underlying liver disease. Extended and multivisceral resections, which have been performed in many patients reported by Pinna et al., are warranted. However, the problem of recurrent disease after liver transplantation if the tumor was advanced cannot be overcome with fibrolamellar carcinoma either. Therefore, we do not consider liver transplantation to be an appropriate treatment for fibrolamellar carcinoma if the patient is noncirrhotic.

Cholangiocarcinoma

Cholangiocarcinoma is an adenocarcinoma arising from the intrahepatic biliary epithelium and developing in noncirrhotic liver. It is commonly divided into the peripheral and hilar types. According to a widely accepted definition of cholangiocarcinoma, only adenocarcinomas of the peripheral type should be classified as cholangiocarcinomas. Peripheral cholangiocarcinoma becomes symptomatic by size as it enlarges.

Unresectable tumors and functional restrictions, but also the assumption that major extirpative procedures might provide an increased chance of a cure, resulted in efforts to resect the entire intrahepatic biliary tree by combining hilar resection, total hepatectomy, and liver transplantation. Arguments in favor of this approach included a putative rise in the rates of formally curative resections and the simultaneous therapy of underlying or associated diseases, e.g., primary sclerosing cholangitis, as well as the prevention of de novo and recurrent tumors, since multifocal lesions within the biliary tract may be identified in as many as 10% of patients. Postoperative mortality was even expected to decrease, since liver transplants in a patient population that does not have complicating portal hypertension are usually fairly straightforward. However, postoperative and long-term survival figures have been disappointing. In a review of 34 patients originating from 13 studies, 90-day mortality and 5-year survival rates after total hepatectomy and liver transplantation for peripheral cholangiocarcinoma were approximately 29% and 6%, respectively [28]. Cancer recurrence predominated as the cause of death in 88% of the patients surviving more than 90 days posttransplant.

Similar results have also been reported for hilar cholangiocarcinoma. Many of these patients underwent operations in the 1980s, when some surgical endeavors were made to establish liver transplantation as a widespread treatment for liver diseases in general. Therefore, postoperative mortality rates were expected to be reduced by at least half some 10 years later. However, the major obstacle to patient longevity still remains the unpredictable risk caused by the potentially accelerated growth of residual tumor cells during chronic immunosuppression. This unfavorable experience is also reflected in a single-center report by Pichlmayr et al. [29] on 18 patients undergoing liver transplantation for cholangiocarcinoma. None of the patients, including four patients with T2 tumors, survived beyond 2 years posttransplant. Disappointing long-term results after abdominal organ cluster transplantation were reported by Alessiani et al. [30, 31]. Among a variety of liver tumors such as endocrine tumors, sarcoma, and HCC, cholangiocarcinoma fared the worst, with a 5-year survival rate of 15%.

References

1. Engstrom PF, McGlynn K, Hoffmann JP (1997) Primary neoplasms of the liver. In: Holland JF, Bast RC, Morton DL, Frei E, Kufe DW, Weichselbaum RR (eds) Cancer medicine, 4th edn. Williams & Wilkins, Baltimore, pp 1923–1938
2. Ortner MA, Liebetruth J, Schreiber S, et al. (1998) Photodynamic therapy of non-resectable cholangiocarcinoma. Gastroenterology 114:536–542
3. Curley SA, Izzo F, Delrio P, et al. (1999) Radiofrequency ablation of unresectable primary and metastatic hepatic malignancies: results in 123 patients. Ann Surg 230:1–8
4. Vogl TJ, Mack MG, Roggan A, et al. (1998) Internally cooled power laser for MR-guided interstitial laser-induced thermotherapy of liver lesions: initial clinical results. Radiology 209:381–385
5. Livraghi T, Goldberg SN, Lazzaroni S, et al. (1999) Small hepatocellular carcinoma: treatment with radio-frequency ablation versus ethanol injection. Radiology 210:655–661
6. Bruix J, Llovet JM, Castells A, et al. (1998) Transarterial embolization versus symptomatic treatment in patients with advanced hepatocellular carcinoma: results of a randomized, controlled trial in a single institution. Hepatology 27:1578–1583
7. Llovet JM, Fuster J, Bruix J. (1999) Intention-to-treat analysis of surgical treatment for early hepatocellular carcinoma: resection versus transplantation. Hepatology 30:1434–1440

8. Lau WY, Leung TW, Ho SK, et al. (1999) Adjuvant intra-arterial iodine-131-labelled lipiodole for resectable hepatocellular carcinoma: a prospective randomised trial. Lancet 353:797–801

9. Jonas S, Bechstein WO, Kling N, et al. (1997) Therapie des primären hepatozellulären Karzinoms. Dtsch Med Wochenschr 122:617–620

10. Belghiti J, Panis Y, Farges O, et al. (1991) Intrahepatic recurrence after resection of hepatocellular carcinoma complicating cirrhosis. Ann Surg 214:114–117

11. Babineau TJ, Lewis WD, Jenkins RL, et al. (1994) Role of staging laparoscopy in the treatment of hepatic malignancy. Am J Surg 167:151–154

12. Lo CM, Lai EC, Liu CL, et al. (1998) Laparoscopy and laparoscopic ultrasonography avoid exploratory laparotomy in patients with hepatocellular carcinoma. Ann Surg 227:527–532

13. Yokoyama I, Carr B, Saitsu H, et al. (1991) Accelerated growth rates of recurrent hepatocellular carcinoma after liver transplantation. Cancer 68:2095–2100

14. Bismuth H, Chiche L, Adam R, et al. (1993) Liver resection versus transplantation for hepatocellular carcinoma in cirrhotic patients. Ann Surg 218:145–151

15. Pichlmayr R, Weimann A, Oldhafer KJ, et al. (1995) Role of liver transplantation in the treatment of unresectable liver cancer. World J Surg 19:807–813

16. Mazzaferro V, Regalia E, Doci R, et al. (1996) Liver transplantation for the treatment of small hepatocellular carcinomas in patients with cirrhosis. N Engl J Med 334:693–699

17. Llovet JM, Bruix J, Fuster J, et al. (1998) Liver transplantation for small hepatocellular carcinoma: the tumor-node-metastasis classification does not have prognostic power. Hepatology 27:1572–1577

18. Jonas S, Bechstein WO, Steinmüller T, et al. (2001) Vascular invasion and histopathological grading determine outcome after liver transplantation for hepatocellular carcinoma in cirrhosis. Hepatology 33:1080–1086

19. Majno PE, Adam R, Bismuth H, et al. (1997) Influence of preoperative transarterial lipiodol chemoembolization on resection and transplantation for hepatocellular carcinoma in patients with cirrhosis. Ann Surg 226:688–701

20. Olthoff KM, Rosove MH, Shackleton CR, et al. (1995) Adjuvant chemotherapy improves survival after liver transplantation for hepatocellular carcinoma. Ann Surg 221:734–741

21. Okuda K, Nakashima T, Kojiro M, et al. (1989) Hepatocellular carcinoma without cirrhosis in Japanese patients. Gastroenterology 97:140–146

22. Bismuth H, Chiche L, Castaing D (1995) Surgical treatment of hepatocellular carcinomas in noncirrhotic liver: experience with 68 liver resections. World J Surg 19:35–41

23. Iwatsuki S, Starzl TE, Sheahan DG, et al. (1991) Hepatic resection versus transplantation for hepatocellular carcinoma. Ann Surg 214:221–228

24. Craig JR, Peters RL, Edmondson HA, et al. (1980) Fibrolamellar carcinoma of the liver: a tumor of adolescents and young adults with distinctive clinico-pathologic features. Cancer 46:372–379

25. Soreide O, Czerniak A, Bradpiece H, et al. (1986) Characteristics of fibrolamellar hepatocellular carcinoma. A study of nine cases and a review of the literature. Am J Surg 151:518–523

26. Berman MA, Burnham JA, Sheahan DG (1988) Fibrolamellar carcinoma of the liver: an immunohistochemical study of nineteen cases and a review of the literature. Hum Pathol 19:784–794

27. Pinna AD, Iwatsuki S, Lee RG, et al. (1997) Treatment of fibrolamellar hepatoma with subtotal hepatectomy or transplantation. Hepatology 26:877–883

28. Curley SA, Levin B, Rich TA (1995) Management of specific malignancies: liver and bile ducts. In: Abeloff MD, Armitage JO, Lichter AS, Niederhuber JE (eds) Clinical Oncology. Churchill Livingstone, New York, pp 1305–1372
29. Pichlmayr R, Lamesch P, Weimann A, et al. (1995) Surgical treatment of cholangio-cellular carcinoma. World J Surg 19:83–88
30. Alessiani M, Tzakis A, Todo S, et al. (1995) Assessment of five-year experience with abdominal cluster transplantation. J Am Coll Surg 180:1–9
31. Starzl TE, Todo S, Tzakis A, et al. (1989) Abdominal organ cluster transplantation for the treatment of upper abdominal malignancies. Ann Surg 210:374–386

Long-Term Results of Transplantation for Hepatocellular Carcinoma With or Without Cirrhosis: 15 Years'-Experience at Paul Brousse Hospital

RENÉ ADAM, DANIEL AZOULAY, DENIS CASTAING, DIDIER SAMUEL, FAOUZI SALIBA, CYRILLE FERAY, ERIC SAVIER, LUC-ANTOINE VEILHAN, PHILIPPE ICHAI, and HENRI BISMUTH

Summary. Hepatocellular carcinoma (HCC) still remains a controversial indication for liver transplantation (LT). An evaluation of long-term results is mandatory to define the patients who are likely to benefit from cadaveric or living-related LT. During 15 years' experience, 220 LTs were performed consecutively at a single institution for HCC in patients with or without underlying cirrhosis (195 and 25 cases, respectively). The patients were younger and the proportion of females was higher in the noncirrhotic group ($P < 0.001$). Perioperative mortality (≤ 2 months) was 4% in cirrhotic and 0% in non cirrhotic patients. In spite of a higher incidence of recurrence related to more extensive tumors in HCC without cirrhosis (54% vs. 20%, $P < 0.001$), survival after transplantation was similar: 60% and 48% at 5 and 10 years, respectively, for patients without cirrhosis, and 73% and 39%, respectively, for patients with underlying cirrhosis (P not significant). While the combination of size and number of tumors was highly predictive of recurrence and survival in the cirrhotic group, this was not the case for non-cirrhotic patients. However, portal invasion was poorly associated with survival in both groups. HCC with and without underlying cirrhosis represents two separate entities with different patterns of evolution. The criteria of selection for transplantation should follow different policies in these two groups of patients.

Key words. Hepatocellular carcinoma, Liver transplantation, Prognosis

Centre Hépato-Biliaire, Hôpital Paul Brousse, Université Paris-Sud, 12–14 Avenue Paul Vaillant Couturier, 94804 Villejuif, France

Introduction

Hepatocellular carcinoma (HCC) is one of the most common malignancies worldwide, accounting for more than one million deaths annually [1]. The current epidemic of cirrhosis due to the hepatitis C virus, with a malignant transformation rate of 2%–8% per year, is leading to a steady increase in the number of new cases [2]. HCC still remains a controversial indication for liver transplantation (LT). The lack of organs has restricted the use of transplantation to patients with a very limited intrahepatic tumor, and excluded those patients with large (>50 mm) and/or multinodular (>3 nodules) HCC [3, 4]. The increasing use of alternatives to cadaveric full-size organs, such as split, domino, or living-related livers, now makes it possible to carry out transplantation in some patients with HCC who would otherwise not meet the conventional criteria for LT. However, an evaluation of the long-term results of LT for HCC is mandatory to define the patients who are likely to benefit from such alternatives. Separate analyses should be made of HCC with and without superimposed cirrhosis, since the indications for transplantation are usually different in the two cases. While the indications are well established for HCC with cirrhosis, they are still pending for cases of HCC without cirrhosis. The present study was conducted to evaluate the long-term results of transplantation for HCC with and without cirrhosis at our institution over a period of 15 years.

Patients and Methods

From December 1984 to December 1999, 1482 LTs were performed consecutively in 1304 patients at our institution. Of these, 220 (14.8%) were for HCC in patients with (195 cases) or without (25 cases of nonfibrolamellar HCC) underlying cirrhosis. For the latter, the first indication was always the tumor, but this was not the case for the former: 47 tumors (24%) were found incidentally either at the pretransplant check-up for end-stage cirrhosis (18 cases), or on pathological examination of the specimen (29 cases). The patients' characteristics and the causes of the underlying cirrhosis are summarized in Table 1.

Patient Selection

HCC with Underlying Cirrhosis

There were two different periods in the selection of patients during these 15 years. During 1985–1991, patients underwent liver transplantation primarily because their tumor was not resectable (too large, multinodular HCC, or poor hepatic function), with the only contraindication being the presence of extrahepatic spread. A comparison of the results of transplantations with those of

TABLE 1. Characteristics of patients transplanted for hepatocellular carcinoma with and without cirrhosis

	Cirrhosis	No cirrhosis	P
No. of patients	195	25	–
Age (mean and range in years)	53.2 (16–69)	38.2 (10–62)	0.0001
Male/female	167/28	15/10	0.001
HbsAg+	43 (22%)	2 (8%)	
VHC+	79 (41%)	–	0.001
HbsAg+ and VHC+	14 (7%)	–	
Cause of cirrhosis			
Primary biliary	5 (3%)		
Virus-related	136 (70%)		
Alcoholic	32 (16%)		
Other	22 (11%)		

HbsAg, hepatitis B surface antigen; VHC, viral hepatitis C

resections during this first period [3] led us to propose transplantation for patients usually treated by partial resection (≤3 nodules and ≤3 cm), and not for patients with large multinodular tumors (>3 and >3 cm). From 1991 to date, selection for cadaveric LT has favored patients with tumors of limited number and size and the absence of portal invasion [5]. However, the selection of patients for alternative techniques to conventional LT, i.e., domino or living-related LT, has been less stringent because these techniques reduce the problem of cadaveric organ shortage. However, portal invasion or the presence of an extrahepatic tumor are still absolute contraindications to a transplant procedure.

HCC Without Underlying Cirrhosis

The selection process for these patients has been uniform during the study period. Liver transplantation was reserved for patients who had a contraindication to a partial resection and in the absence of extrahepatic disease or portal invasion by the tumor.

Preoperative Management

Pretransplant assessment included the staging of intrahepatic disease by liver ultrasound (US) examination, abdominal computed tomography (CT), and at least one course of transarterial chemoembolization (TACE) in those patients who did not have Child stage C cirrhosis. The search for any extrahepatic tumors included chest CT and a radionuclide bone scan.

A pretransplant treatment of HCC was performed in most cirrhotic patients, mainly those with known tumors, either by TACE (108 patients, 55%), liver resection (15 patients, 8%), or liver-directed therapies (alcohol injection, cryotherapy, radiofrequency, 13 patients, 6%). In noncirrhotic patients, TACE was performed in 15 patients (40%), and a preliminary liver resection was performed in 6 patients (21%).

Operative Technique

The operative technique has been described extensively in previous reports [3, 5]. In brief, the transplant operation is started with a limited right subcostal incision, and a full exploration of the abdominal cavity looking for possible contraindications. Lymph nodes of the hepatic pedicle or of the celiac region are systematically resected, as well as any suspect peritoneal deposit, for frozen-section examination. We proceed with the liver transplantation only in the absence of any extrahepatic tumor, or of a tumor thrombus in the portal system. A cell saver is not used to decrease the risk of disseminating tumor cells that may be shed during manipulation of the liver. When tumor nodules are located close to the retrohepatic vena cava, this is resected with the whole liver to achieve better tumor clearance.

Postoperative Care

Chemotherapy was administered in the presence of adverse histologic features (tumors >3, size >30 mm, microvascular invasion, satellite nodules, absence or invaded tumor capsule) for a total of nine courses, unless complications impeded its administration. Alpha-fetoprotein measurements and liver US scans were performed every 3 months, and abdominal and chest CT scans were performed every 6 months, with a radionuclide bone scan performed if these was any clinical suspicion of bone metastasis.

Results

Perioperative Mortality

Eight patients (3.6%) died within 2 months after liver transplantation. All were in the cirrhotic group. The mortality was therefore 4% for cirrhotic patients (8/195) and nil (0/28) for noncirrhotic patients. There were one intraoperative death from cardiac arrhythmia and seven postoperative deaths from early postoperative cardiac failure (1), sepsis complicating graft dysfunction (1), retransplantation for primary nonfunction (1), bacterial sepsis with shock (2), and diffuse aspergillosis (2).

Morbidity

Among the major complications, there were 12 cases of postoperative bleeding (5%), 7 hepatic arterial thromboses (3%), 2 portal thromboses (1%), 3 biliary fistulas (1%), 7 cases of intraabdominal bile leakage (3%), and 17 biliary stenoses (8%). Fourteen patients needed a retransplantation (6%), of which 3 were for primary nonfunction.

Tumor Recurrence

After a mean follow-up of 57.7 months (range 3–182 months), 39 patients (20%) had a recurrence in the cirrhotic group; 14 recurrences (56%) were observed in the noncirrhotic group after a mean follow-up of 63.3 months (range 3–142 months). The liver and lungs were the most common sites of recurrence (Table 2), and they occurred mainly within the first 2 years following LT (77% and 67% of recurrences, respectively). While the combination of the size and number of tumors was highly predictive of recurrence in the cirrhotic group ($P = 0.0005$), this was not the case for noncirrhotic patients ($P = 0.41$) (Table 2). Repeat surgical procedures were performed to resect the tumoral recurrence in 10% of patients (4/39) in the cirrhotic group (2 hepatectomies, 1 right adrenalectomy, 1 resection of a bone metastasis), and in 50% of patients (7/14) in the noncirrhotic group (1 hepatectomy, 4 pulmonary resections, 1 resection of a bone metastasis).

Of 39 and 14 patients in whom HCC recurred in the cirrhotic and noncirrhotic group, respectively, 33 (85%) and 9 (64%), respectively, died of metastatic disease. As of June 2001, 6 cirrhotic and 5 noncirrhotic patients who experienced recurrence were still alive, and of these, 1 and 3, respectively, had survived for 5 years from the first recurrence.

TABLE 2. Tumor recurrence after liver transplantation for hepatocellular carcinoma with and without cirrhosis

	Cirrhosis	No cirrhosis	P
No of patients	195	25	–
Follow-up (months)	57.7 (3–182)	63.3 (3–142)	NS
Overall recurrence	39 (20%)	14 (56%)	0.001
Recurrence nonincidental	38/143 (27%)	14 (56%)	0.01
Primary site of recurrence			
Liver	10 (26%)	1 (7%)	
Lungs	9 (23%)	7 (50%)	
Bone	8 (21%)	4 (29%)	
Other	12 (30%)	3 (21%)	
Recurrence vs. no. and size			
≤3 ≤30 mm	7/103 (7%)	1/4 (25%)	NS
≤3 >30 mm	11/37 (30%)	3/7 (43%)	NS
>3 ≤30 mm	8/26 (31%)	4/5 (80%)	0.04
>3 >30 mm	12/27 (44%)	6/9 (67%)	NS
	$P = 0.0005$	$P = 0.41$	

NS, not significant

Survival Rates

The overall survival rate for the whole group of patients transplanted for HCC was 62% at 5 years and 46% at 10 years. Survival was 60% and 48%, respectively, for patients with underlying cirrhosis, and 73% and 42%, respectively, for those without cirrhosis (*P* not significant) (Fig. 1). The disease-free survival rate was increased in the cirrhotic compared with the noncirrhotic group (60% vs. 36% at 5 years, and 48% vs. 19% at 10 years; *P* = 0.03). At the end of the study period, 106 patients (54%) and 9 patients (36%) were alive and free of disease in the cirrhotic and the noncirrhotic groups, respectively.

Prognostic Factors for Survival (Table 3)

Patients with HCC and cirrhosis with multinodular tumors (>3 nodules on pathological examination of the specimen) had significantly lower survival rates than those with paucinodular HCC (42% vs. 65%, respectively, at 5 years; *P* = 0.01). In addition, large tumors (>3 cm) were associated with a decreased survival rate compared with smaller tumors (41% vs. 69%, *P* < 0.01). However, patients with HCC of 30–50 mm had no better outcome than those with tumors >50 mm (43% vs. 40%). In contrast, in patients without underlying cirrhosis neither the multinodularity (69% vs. 100%, *P* not significant) nor the large size of the HCC (78% vs. 67%, *P* not significant) had a negative influence on the 5-year survival rate. Accordingly, while the combination the

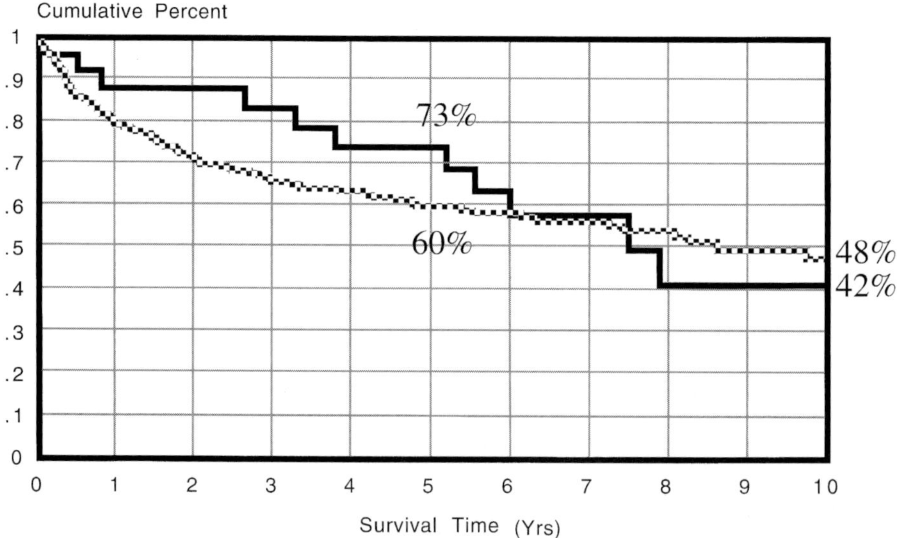

FIG. 1. Survival after liver transplantation for HCC with and without underlying cirrhosis. *Black line*, no cirrhosis; *broken line*, with cirrhosis. *P* not significant

TABLE 3. Five- and 10-year survival rates after liver transplantation for HCC according to the presence of underlying cirrhosis and the characteristics of the tumor

	Cirrhosis (195 patients)		Noncirrhosis (25 patients)	
	5 years	10 years	5 years	10 years
Overall	61	48	74	40
Tumor size				
≤30 mm	69	62	67	–
30–50 mm	43	31	80	80
>50 mm	40	15	78	31
Number of nodules				
1	72	70	100	–
2–3	58	35	50	25
>3	42	33	69	37
Number + size				
≤3 ≤30 mm	73	65	75	–
≤3 >30 mm	46	20	83	67
>3 ≤30 mm	51	43	60	–
>3 >30 mm	35	25	74	37
Portal invasion				
Yes	25	0	51	–
No	66	54	81	46
Microvascular invasion				
Yes	47	33	59	25
No	70	59	86	–

number and the maximal size of tumors was closely related to survival following transplantation for HCC with underlying cirrhosis (73% at 5 years for patients with lesions ≤3≤30 mm vs. 35% for those with lesions >3>30 mm, $P < 0.01$), this was not the case for HCC without cirrhosis (75% vs. 74%, respectively, for the same groups of patients; P not significant). Portal invasion as assessed by histology was poorly associated with survival for both forms of HCC with and without cirrhosis (25% in patients with portal invasion vs. 66% in patients with no portal invasion in the cirrhotic group, $P < 0.01$; 51% vs. 81%, respectively, $P = 0.09$, in the noncirrhotic group). Microvascular invasion was also associated with a poor prognosis in cirrhotic (47% vs. 70% 5-year survival) and in noncirrhotic (59% vs. 86%) patients. Surgical treatment of the recurrence following LT improved survival as compared with that of patients with nonoperable recurrence, and this improvement was greater in previously cirrhotic patients (60% vs. 12% at 5 years, $P < 0.01$). In noncirrhotic patients, survival tended to be improved but the difference was not significant (75% vs. 55%).

Discussion

The results of this study demonstrate that HCC with and without underlying cirrhosis represents two separate entities with different patterns of evolution. Patients without cirrhosis are younger and the proportion of females is significantly higher compared with the cirrhotic group. In spite of a higher incidence of recurrence related to more extensive tumors in patients with HCC without cirrhosis, the long-term survival after transplantation is similar, and in some cases even better, than that of patients with HCC with cirrhosis. This is particularly true for tumors >30 mm and/or multinodular (>3), which show 5-year survival rates exceeding 70%, while survival is only 35% to 51% in patients with underlying cirrhosis. The reason why such a difference appears remains to be elucidated. The absence of perioperative mortality in transplantation in noncirrhotic patients compared with the rate of 4% in patients with HCC and underlying cirrhosis may be part of the explanation. Also, the higher rate of resecting tumoral recurrence in patients transplanted for HCC without cirrhosis (50% vs. only 10% of HCC with cirrhosis) could partially explain the good outcome of these patients, since it is known that surgery, when possible, improves the outcome. However, different aspects of tumor biology and tumor growth could act as critical factors between these two entities. Conflicting results have been reported in the literature, but these are probably related to different patient selection criteria. While Pichlmayr et al. [6] found no difference in the survival of patients with and without cirrhosis, O'Grady et al. [7] observed a better outcome in cirrhotic patients, and Haug et al. [8] showed a better outcome in noncirrhotic patients.

No matter which factors are involved, our results validate the use of less stringent selection criteria for transplantation for tumors without cirrhosis. Currently, noncirrhotic patients only receive a transplant if they have advanced nonresectable HCC, while patients with HCC with nodules which are limited in size and number are routinely transplanted in the presence of cirrhosis.

Many studies, including ours, have reported on the results of transplantation for HCC in patients with cirrhosis [3–15]. Our present data on the main influence of the number, the maximum size, and the vascular invasion of tumors relate to our published reports. However, in contrast to reports on tumor size which argue for a prognostic cut-off at 5 cm [4, 9–12], our results clearly indicate that 3 cm is the realistic limit of prognostic significance. The 5-year survival rates were very similar for the groups of HCC of 3–5 cm or >5 cm in size (43% and 40%, respectively), but they were significantly lower than that of HCC ≤3 cm (69%). The use of the combined number and maximal size of the tumors, each with a cut-off value of 3, gives a good prognostic estimation of long-term survival. It is also of much more practical use than the usual TNM classification which does not predict the outcome as well [11, 12].

Our criteria facilitate the selection of patients for transplantation. While large multinodular HCC (>3, >30 mm) should logically be excluded from transplantation (5-year survival 35%) and small HCC with few nodules (≤3, ≤30 mm) remain the ideal indication, the in-between groups of patients who are usually excluded from cadaveric LT because of isolated multinodularity (>3) or isolated large tumor size (>30 mm) still have 5-year survival rates of 51% and 46%, respectively. In our view, this is a reason for considering these patients for transplantation using split, domino, or living related-donor organs. In contrast, portal invasion by the tumor, irrespective of the proximal or distal location of the thrombus, should remain an absolute contraindication, even with the use of alternative techniques to cadaveric LT, given the poor survival rate achieved in this group (25% at 5 years) and the known poor prognosis of microvascular invasion at histology [13].

Fewer series have been published in relation to HCC without cirrhosis [6–8, 14–17]. In spite of a high incidence of tumor recurrences (52%), the survival rates of 74% at 5 years and 40% at 10 years in our series obviously contrast with those in previous reports, which suggested that most patients died of recurrent malignancy within 2 years [7, 14, 16]. The Tumor Registry data also reported a 5-year overall survival rate of only 18% in patients with advanced HCC treated by transplantation [18]. A recent analysis of 16 series reported in the literature has shown that transplantation for HCC without underlying cirrhosis had only a small chance of cure, undoubtedly because of the advanced stages of the cancers [17]. The 5-year survival of 77 patients without cirrhosis who underwent transplantation for HCC was only 11.2%. These poor results were possibly related to a learning curve in terms of the selection process, and some of these patients would probably be excluded from transplantation today because of lymph node or portal invasion by the tumor. In the European Liver Transplant Registry, the survival rate of 415 patients up to June 2000 was 42% at 5 years and 34% at 10 years, which is a better reflection of the current outcome of such patients [19]. If split, domino, or living-related LT brings a change in the spectrum of HCC without cirrhosis it will not be by extending the indications for transplantation since, in contrast to HCC with cirrhosis, it is usual to propose liver replacement for advanced forms of tumor. However, these alternatives to conventional transplantation should significantly reduce the waiting time before grafting, allowing patients who are now rejected from the list to be transplanted "on time," and possibly providing lower rates of recurrence by avoiding tumor spread.

References

1. Loetze MFJ, Carr B (1993) Hepatobiliary neoplasms. Lippincott, Philadelphia
2. Ganne-Carié N, Chastang C, Chapel F, et al. (1996) Predictive score for the development of hepatocellular carcinoma and additional value of live large cell dysplasia in Western patients with cirrhosis. Hepatology 23:1112–1118

3. Bismuth H, Chiche L, Adam R, et al. (1993) Liver resection versus transplantation for hepatocellular carcinoma in cirrhotic patients. Ann Surg 218:145–151

4. Mazzaferro V, Regalia E, Doci R, et al. (1996) Liver transplantation for the treatment of small hepatocellular carcinomas in patients with cirrhosis. N Engl J Med 334: 693–699

5. Adam R, Castaing D, Azoulay D, et al. (1998) Transplantation pour carcinome hepatocellulaire. Ann Chir 52:547–557

6. Pichlmayr R, Weimann A, Oldhafer KJ, et al. (1995) Role of liver transplantation in the treatment of unresectable liver cancer. World J Surg 19:807–813

7. O'Grady JG, Polson RJ, Rolles K, et al. (1988) Liver transplantation for malignant disease: results in 93 consecutive patients. Ann Surg 4:373–379

8. Haug CE, Jenkins RL, Rohrer RJ (1992) Liver transplantation for primary hepatic cancer. Transplantation 53:376

9. Ojogho ON, So SKS, Keefe EB, et al. (1996) Orthotopic liver transplantation for hepatocellular carcinoma. Arch Surg 131:935–941

10. Figueras J, Jaurieta E, Valls C, et al. (1997) Survival after liver transplantation in cirrhotic patients with and without hepatocellular carcinoma: a comparative study. Hepatology 25:1485–1490

11. Llovet JM, Bruix J, Fuster J, et al. (1998) Liver transplantation for small hepatocellular carcinoma. The tumor-node-metastases classification does not have prognostic power. Hepatology 27:1572–1577

12. Mc Peake Jr, O'Grady JG, Zaman S, et al. (1993) Liver transplantation for primary hepatocellular carcinoma: tumor size and number determines outcome. J Hepatol 18: 226–234

13. Hemming AW, Cattral MS, Reed A, et al. (2001) Liver transplantation for hepatocellular carcinoma. Ann Surg 233:652–659

14. Iwatsuki S, Klintmalm GBG, Starzl TE (1982) Total hepatectomy and liver replacement (orthotopic liver transplantation) for primary hepatic malignancy. World J Surg 6: 81–85

15. Iwatsuki S, Starzl TE, Sheahan DG, et al. (1991) Hepatic resection versus transplantation for hepatocellular carcinoma. Ann Surg 214:221–229

16. Ringe B, Pichlmayr R, Wittekind C, et al. (1991) Surgical treatment of hepatocellular carcinoma: experience with liver resection and transplantation in 198 patients. World J Surg 15:270–285

17. Houben KW, McCall JL (1999) Liver transplantation for hepatocellular carcinoma in patients without underlying disease. A systematic review. Liver Transplant Surg 5: 91–95

18. Penn I (1991) Hepatic transplantation for primary and metastatic cancers of the liver. Surgery 110:726–735

19. European Liver Transplant Registry (ELTR) (2000) Statistical analysis of liver transplantation in Europe. Update, December 2000

Living Donor Liver Transplantation for Malignant Hepatic Tumors

Koichi Tanaka

A program of living donor liver transplantation was in operation for patients with malignant hepatic tumors. Since then there have been many controversies concerning indications based on tumor stage, the immunosuppressive regimens, postoperative chemotherapy, and preoperative ablation treatment. Between February 1999 and January 2001 a series of 30 patients with hepatocellular carcinoma received living donor liver transplants. The criteria for inclusion in this group were no evidence of extrahepatic tumor and no evidence of macroscopic tumor involvement in the portal or hepatic veins. The number or size of the tumor(s) was not taken into consideration. The patients consisted of 22 males and 8 females with a mean age of 49 years (range 12–68 years). The underlying liver diseases were hepatitis C ($n = 12$), hepatitis B ($n = 11$), hepatitis C and B ($n = 2$), alcoholism ($n = 1$), citrullinemia ($n = 1$), and unknown ($n = 3$). There was 1 patient in stage I, 3 in stage II, 3 in stage III, and 22 in stage IVA, as determined by preoperative imaging examinations. Immunosuppression consisted of tacrolimus monotherapy. To assess tumor recurrence, the α-feto protein and protein induced by vitamin K absence or antagonism (PIVKA-II) levels were checked monthly; and CT scans (abdomen, chest, brain) and bone scimtigraphy were undertaken every 3 months. Eight recipients died of sepsis ($n = 3$), peritonitis ($n = 2$), pneumonia ($n = 1$), cereberal bleeding ($n = 1$), and asphyxia ($n = 1$). Of 22 surviving recipients, 2 had recurrence of the tumor (one with lung metastasis and tumor in the diaphragm, one with brain metastasis) during the mean follow-up period of 9 months. We concluded that further long-term follow-up is necessary to evaluate the efficacy of living donor liver transplantation for patients with hepatocellular carcinoma.

Department of Transplantation and Immunology, Kyoto University Graduate School of Medicine, Kyoto, Japan

Part 5
Novel Strategies in Immunosuppression

Optimizing the Use of Neoral in Liver and Kidney Transplantation by C_2 Monitoring

GARY A. LEVY

Summary. Neoral absorption profiling is a concept in therapeutic drug monitoring (TDM) designed to optimize further the clinical benefits in transplant patients. A single blood-level measurement 2 h after dosing (C_2), has been shown to be a significantly more accurate predictor of drug exposure in both live and kidney transplant patients than trough levels, and its use results in a reduction in the incidence and severity of cellular rejection. In maintenance liver transplant recipients, the adoption of C_2 monitoring defines patients who are both over- and underdosed, which is not distinguished by C_0 (trough) measurements. Further adjustments of C_2 levels to recommended targets, even at 5 and 10 years posttransplant, results in improvements in nephrotoxicity without exposing the patient to the risk of rejection.

In a prospective trial in de novo renal transplant recipients, patients who achieved target area under the concentration-time curve (AUC) levels of 4500–5500 ng·h/ml within 5 days of transplant had an incidence of acute cellular rejection of 7% compared with 37% rejection in those patients who did not achieve this target level. Of the single-sample points, C_2 correlates best with AUC_{0-4} ($r^2 = 0.86$); C_0 had the poorest correlation. In an international study in 21 centers examining absorption profiling, C_2 samples were the most accurate predictors of AUC_{0-4} and freedom from rejection.

Despite a level of simplicity comparable to a trough-level measurement, Neoral absorption profiling, and specifically measurement of 2-h postdose levels (C_2), is a much more sensitive approach to assessing the pharmacokinetics and predicting the clinical impact of Neoral in the individual patient, resulting in a marked reduction in the incidence of acute cellular rejection and improved long-term graft function.

Multi-Organ Transplantation, Toronto General Hospital, 621 University Avenue, 10th Floor, Suite 116, Toronto, Ontario M5G 2C4, Canada

Key words. Cyclosporine, Transplant, Kidney, Liver, Drug monitoring

Introduction

There has been renewed interest in the development of more effective therapeutic monitoring tools for optimizing cyclosporin A (CsA) immuno-suppression than predose "trough" (or C_0) concentrations [1–3]. There is evidence that C_0 does not accurately reflect an individual's CsA exposure [2, 4, 5]. Recent evidence suggests that the most sensitive marker for extent and consistency of CsA exposure exists within the absorption phase in the individual transplant patient (Fig. 1) [1, 6, 7].

The absorption phase for CsA occurs around the first 4 h after the administration of Neoral (Novartis Pharma A.G., Basel, Switzerland) and is characterized by rapid changes in blood CsA concentrations and a high degree of interpatient and intrapatient variability [6]. More importantly, this phase reflects the patient's capacity to absorb CsA from the gastrointestinal tract, which is dependent on concurrent medications and the integrity of the gastrointestinal tract [8]. Therefore, the advances in therapeutic drug monitoring (TDM) methods that provide estimations of CsA absorption appear to provide useful predictive information about an individual patient's outcome, at least in the short term. CsA absorption markers may provide greater precision in the optimization of Neoral dosing in the transplant recipient.

The goal of this review is to provide a more comprehensive understanding of the absorption profiling–monitoring strategy that has been developed to optimize Neoral dosing in liver and renal transplant recipients, and how it has evolved into the use of a single sampling point at 2 h postdose (C_2) [1, 7].

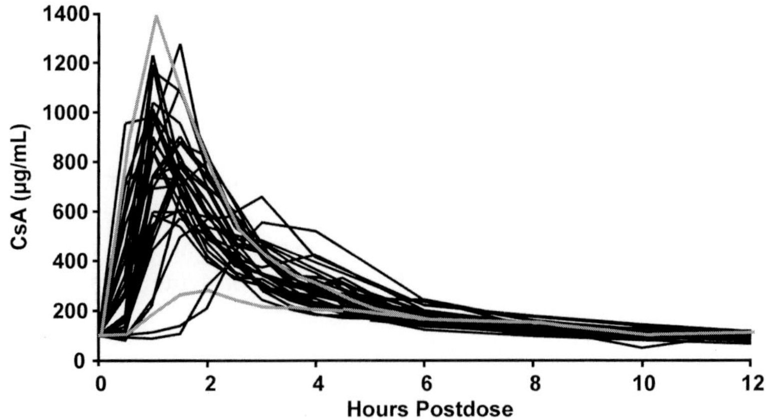

FIG. 1. Interpatient variability of cyclosporin A (*CsA*) absorption is not captured by C_0. Patient differences are highlighted in the absorption phase (adapted from Johnston et al. [6])

The first steps towards the development of a more precise monitoring strategy for CsA resulted from studies by Kahan and co-workers [4, 9] that identified a link between the pharmacokinetics of CsA and clinical outcomes in individual transplant recipients. The area under the concentration–time curve (AUC) for CsA over a 12-h dosing interval was a more precise predictor of graft loss and the incidence of acute rejection than other parameters, including the predose trough concentration [4]. This conclusion was supported by an independent study by First and colleagues [5], who also found a direct correlation between AUC and acute rejection incidence in renal transplant recipients in the first 12 months posttransplant. These studies not only identified the CsA AUC as a sensitive predictor of outcomes, but also reinforced the lack of predictability of C_0 concentrations. Although predose trough concentrations continued to be used as the established monitoring tool in optimizing the dosing of CsA, the evidence was clear that patient outcomes could be improved with the adoption of alternative TDM methods.

Subsequent studies on CsA pharmacokinetics in renal transplant patients identified intrapatient variability in AUC values over time as correlating directly with the risk of chronic rejection (Fig. 2) [9, 10]. This evidence provided the rationale to develop new monitoring strategies based on the AUC, or the total drug exposure that the patient had received over a dosing interval. A major challenge to the acceptance of this more extensive monitoring strategy was the impracticality, and the added expense of obtaining and processing multiple blood samples for the determination of the AUC value. In addition, the effort required in monitoring patients with the AUC strategy probably contributed to its lack of widespread acceptance in the transplant community.

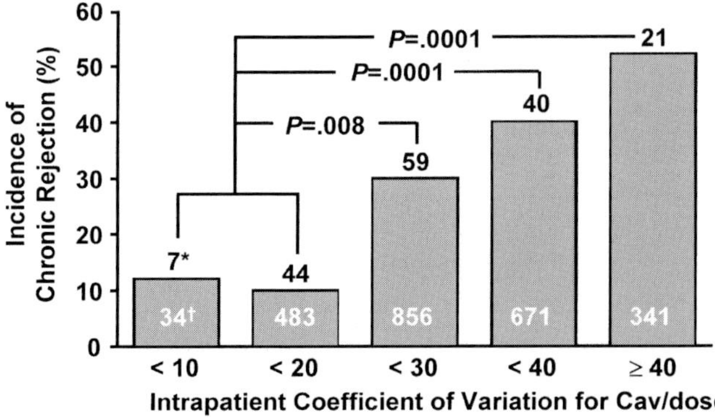

FIG. 2. Variability in CsA exposure increases the risk of chronic rejection (adapted from Kahan et al. [9]). *Number of patients. †Number of pharmacokinetic determinations

This was overcome by the introduction of the sparse-sampling algorithm for the estimation of AUC values by the use of as few as two or three blood samples over the CsA dosing interval. This concept was introduced by Atholl Johnston (St. Bartholomew's Hospital, London, UK) and promoted as a practical TDM tool in clinical practice by Kahan and colleagues [11, 12]. The CsA concentration values were inserted into the appropriate place in a weighted equation specific for an analytical method and a particular patient population. The solution provided an accurate estimate of the AUC for the dosing interval.

Rationale for Utilizing CsA Absorption Profiling

A pharmacokinetic analysis of CsA variability in renal and cardiac transplant recipients identified the absorption phase as the area of greatest interpatient and intrapatient variability [6]. For example, in renal transplant recipients, intrapatient variability was 22% at C_2, and dropped to around 5% from 4 to 12h postdose. Interpatient variability was greatest in the first 2h postdose (range 42%–53%), and stabilized to around 35% from 4 to 12h postdose. Similar results were obtained from the pharmacokinetic variability analysis of data in de novo cardiac transplant recipients. Two other studies have demonstrated that the pharmacodynamic effects of CsA are maximal and most consistent around the peak absorption time postdose, which is between the 1.5- and 2.5-h points. Halloran and colleagues [13] measured the extent of calcineurin inhibition (the primary immunosuppressive mechanism of CsA) and its relationship to CsA blood levels. The degree of calcineurin inhibition matched the concentration of CsA in the blood, and the maximal degree of inhibition occurred around 2h postdose. In a second study [14], the percentage of T cells in the peripheral blood activated by interleukin (IL)-2 was significantly reduced at 2h postdose as compared with predose trough (C_0) levels (10% vs. 39% for C_2 and C_0, respectively, $P < 0.05$). These two studies support the concept that the absorption phase represents a potentially valuable approach to optimizing the immunosuppressive effect of CsA, and the search for new monitoring tools may need to focus on the individual patient's profile in the first few hours postdose.

CsA Monitoring Using Absorption Profiling

The Canadian Neoral Formulation Study (NOF-9) multicenter study comparing the two cyclosporine preparations Neoral and Sandimmune in approximately 2000 renal transplant recipients used CsA monitoring by absorption profiling to document CsA drug exposure from the two formulations. A partial AUC value was generated from sampling points in the first 4h postdose and compared with full AUC values in a cohort of the study population [15]. This study invited a reevaluation of the relevance of the full AUC as the definitive TDM tool for optimizing Neoral dosing in transplant patients.

A renal transplant group in Halifax, Nova Scotia, Canada, investigated the potential role of the limited AUC for the first 4 h postdose (AUC_{0-4}) as a monitoring tool to optimize CsA (Neoral) therapy [2, 16]. Their investigations were divided into two phases: a retrospective analysis to determine the sensitivity of AUC_{0-4} as a predictor of outcomes, and a prospective study to test AUC_{0-4} in clinical practice. The retrospective study [2] was completed in 156 de novo renal transplant recipients who were managed on CsA-based triple immuno-suppressive therapy. CsA doses were individualized for each patient by the use of predose trough (C_0) blood-level monitoring, and a pharmacokinetic analy-sis to obtain AUC_{0-4} was completed within the first 7 days after CsA oral therapy was initiated. At 3 months posttransplant, both C_0 and AUC_{0-4} values for each patient were correlated with the incidence of acute rejection episodes (0–3 months) to determine the sensitivity of these monitoring methods to predict clinical events. Acute renal dysfunction (defined as a 30% rise in serum creatinine that was subsequently reduced by lowering the CsA dose) was used as a second clinical-outcomes marker for correlation with C_0 and AUC_{0-4}.

The mean C_0 value for the patients who experienced an acute rejection in the first 3 months was 293 ng/ml, which was identical to the mean C_0 value (294 ng/ml) for the patients who were rejection free (Fig. 3). However, the mean C_0 value for patients who experienced acute renal dysfunction was sig-nificantly higher than that for the patient group who did not experience renal dysfunction. The AUC_{0-4} was a more sensitive predictor of the incidence of both acute rejection and acute renal dysfunction. When patients were placed into three cohorts based on the range of AUC_{0-4} values, a target range between 4400 ng·h/ml and 5500 ng·h/ml was identified that correlated with the lowest incidence of acute rejection and acute renal dysfunction. Patients with an AUC_{0-4} of less than 4400 ng·h/ml ($n = 73$) had an acute rejection incidence of 38% at 3 months posttransplant, compared with an incidence of 7% in the patient group ($n = 30$) who had achieved an AUC_{0-4} within the range of 4400 ng·h/ml to 5500 ng·h/ml by day 5 posttransplant (Fig. 4). Similarly, acute renal dysfunction incidence in the first 3 months was lowest (6%) in the group that achieved AUC_{0-4} levels within the range of 4400 ng·h/ml to 5500 ng·h/ml, and was significantly increased in the group with AUC_{0-4} levels greater than 5500 ng·h/ml (33%; $P < 0.01$). This study demonstrated both the poor predic-tive performance of C_0 and the sensitivity of AUC_{0-4} as a predictor of acute rejections as well as acute renal dysfunction in the de novo renal transplant recipient. This study also identified the AUC_{0-4} target range of 4400 ng·h/ml to 5500 ng·h/ml as potentially the range for achieving optimal immuno-suppression with CsA therapy.

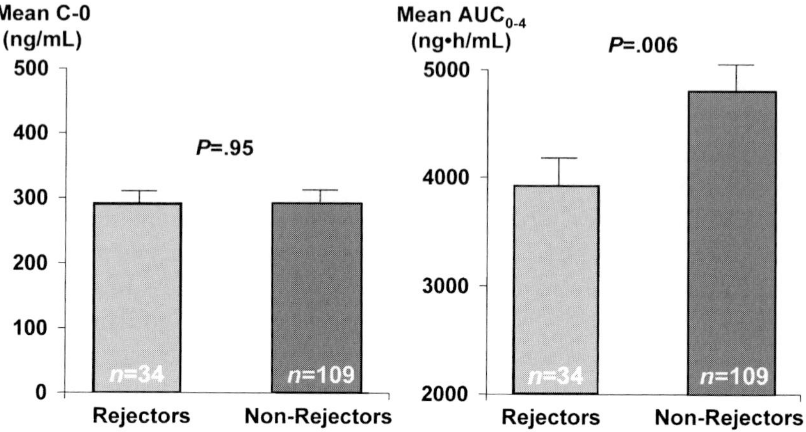

FIG. 3. C_0 does not predict acute rejection, while AUC_{0-4} does (adapted from Mahalati et al. [2])

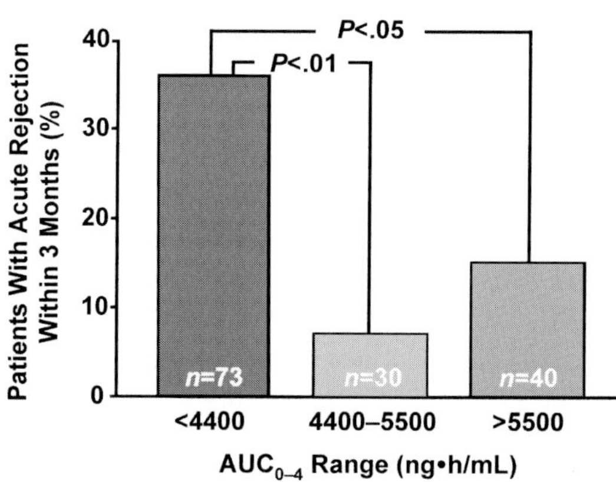

FIG. 4. Optimal AUC_{0-4} range to minimize the risk of acute rejection: 4400–5500 ng·h/ml (adapted from Mahalati et al. [2])

The prospective study [16], completed in 89 de novo renal transplant recipients, was designed to test the AUC_{0-4} monitoring strategy using a desired target range between 4400 ng·h/ml and 5500 ng·h/ml to achieve the optimal Neoral dose in the individual patient. All patients received CsA-based triple immunosuppression, and doses were adjusted with the goal of achieving the target range as soon as possible following transplant. Dose adjustments were made according to the formula:

$$\text{New dose} = \frac{\text{Current dose} \times 5000}{\text{Current } AUC_{0-4}}.$$

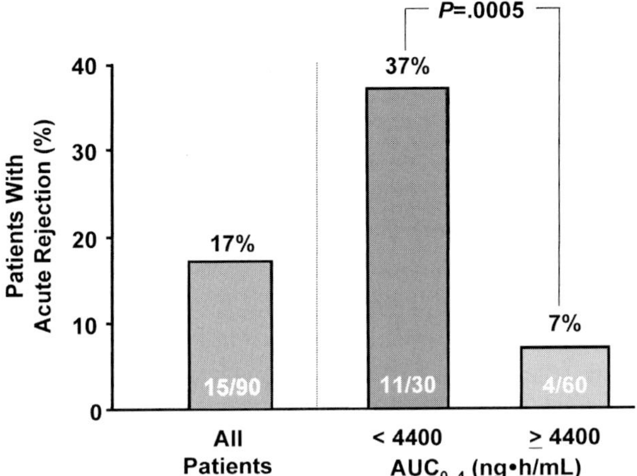

FIG. 5. Achieving target AUC$_{0-4}$ range before day 5 significantly lowers the incidence of acute rejection in the first 6 months (compiled from data from Mahalati et al. [16])

At 6 months posttransplant, the acute rejection incidence was 17% (15/90), and only four patients who rejected their transplant had AUC$_{0-4}$ levels within the target range. Within the population of rejectors ($n = 15$), 11 patients had AUC$_{0-4}$ levels less than 4400 ng·h/ml (Fig. 5). A multivariate analysis identified three statistically significant factors that correlated with acute rejection incidence (AUC$_{0-4}$ level on day 3, $P = 0.0001$; AUC$_{0-4}$ level on day 5, $P = 0.0044$; delayed graft function, $P = 0.015$). The other factors, including C$_0$ level, other immunosuppressants, panel-reactive antibodies, and CsA dose, did not emerge as factors affecting acute rejection incidence. Mean serum creatinine values for the two groups (with AUC$_{0-4}$ less or greater than 4400 ng·h/ml were significantly higher in the low-AUC$_{0-4}$ group (172 ± 54 vs. 127 ± 41 μmol/l for the high-AUC$_{0-4}$ group, $P = 0.001$).

Evolution of C$_2$ Monitoring in Renal Transplantation

AUC$_{0-4}$ monitoring is a sensitive tool used to optimize CsA immunosuppression in renal transplant recipients. However, the tool is not practical in the clinical setting because of three drawbacks: it requires multiple sampling of blood for the determination of AUC$_{0-4}$; the actual value requires a mathematical calculation step; and the test may be too expensive for many clinical hospitals or institutions because of the use of additional costly laboratory tests for CsA levels and the subsequent increase in workload. Therefore, the search for a single blood-sampling point that best reflects the sensitivity of AUC$_{0-4}$

was the focus of several research initiatives that resulted in a broad approval for C_2 monitoring [7].

Two studies in particular completed subanalyses of pharmacokinetic profiles for CsA in de novo renal patients and provided strong evidence for C_2 as the sampling point of choice. Both studies demonstrated that C_2 was a sensitive and accurate surrogate marker of AUC_{0-4} in the de novo patient from the first week to 6 months postinitiation of CsA dosing. The Canadian study [15] was conducted in six renal transplantation centers. De novo subjects ($n = 38$) were followed for 28 days posttransplant, and pharmacokinetic analyses were completed at days 3, 7, and 14 using monoclonal radioimmunoassay (mRIA) analysis for CsA levels. Clinical endpoints (acute rejection, infection, and other adverse events) were assessed on days 3, 7, 14, and 28. The pharmacokinetics of CsA and outcomes analysis demonstrated that AUC_{0-4} correlated significantly with graft rejection ($P = 0.04$). Further analysis showed that C_2 had the best single-point correlation with AUC_{0-4} ($r^2 > 0.8$ for all three time-points) and C_0 had the worst correlation ($r^2 < 0.5$ for all time-points). Furthermore, there was some preliminary clinical evidence to support the use of C_2 as a monitoring tool in de novo renal patients. Mean C_2 ($\pm$ SD) on day 7 for the group who was rejection free ($n = 26$) was 1852 ± 522 ng/ml versus 1116 ± 183 ng/ml ($P < 0.0001$) for the group who experienced a rejection ($n = 10$) by day 28. Patients who achieved a C_2 level above 1500 ng/ml (or 1.5 µg/ml) by day 7 posttransplant did not experience a rejection episode, compared with a 58% incidence of rejection in the group who did not achieve a target of 1.5 µg/ml by day 7 (Fig. 6) using mRIA analysis.

The second study was an open-label, randomized, parallel-group design to investigate the implementation of sparse-sample monitoring for optimizing CsA therapy in comparison with traditional C_0 monitoring. This study was conducted in 204 de novo renal transplant recipients in 20 transplant centers in eight countries. Patients were monitored closely for 90 days, and CsA pharmacokinetics were correlated with clinical outcomes. As in the Canadian study, the best single sampling point that reflects AUC_{0-4} is C_2 ($r^2 = 0.85$), rather than C_0 ($r^2 = 0.12$) or C_3 ($r^2 = 0.70$) [17]. By subdivision of patients into three absorption status levels (low, medium, high) based on dose-normalized C_2 values, there was a clear trend of C_2 levels correlating with the probability of freedom from rejection. When target C_2 levels were >1.7 µg/ml on day 3 in the poor-absorber group, the probability of being rejection-free at 3 months was around 80% compared with 60% for those poor absorbers with a day 3 target of 1.0 µg/ml. This study was not designed to demonstrate the utility of C_2 monitoring, but a subanalysis of the pharmacokinetic data identified C_2 as the most predictive single-point measure of CsA absorption. The target C_2 threshold of 1.7 µg/ml (mRIA analysis) was also identified as providing optimal immunosuppression in the de novo patient in the first 2 weeks posttransplant.

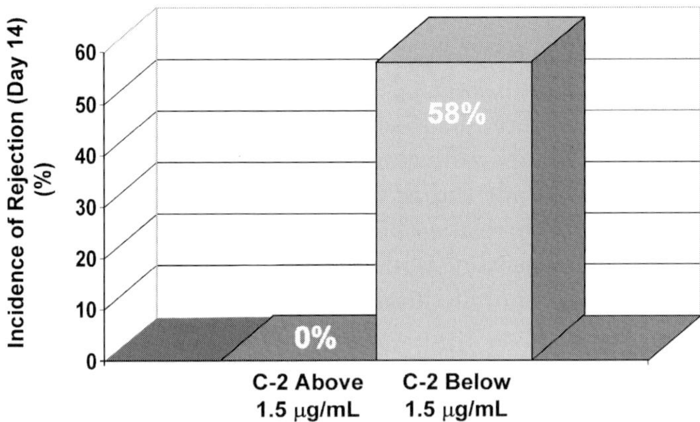

FIG. 6. C$_2$ level at day 7 posttransplant has a significant impact on acute rejection at day 14 [15]

The conclusion of this study was that C$_2$ monitoring is a simple and practical approach to identifying the absorption of CsA in renal transplantation.

C$_2$ in Liver Transplantation

C$_2$ monitoring in liver transplantation has been tested at the Toronto General Hospital as the standard CsA-monitoring procedure in more than 200 de novo patients [3]. Target levels were validated in an international multicenter trial specifically designed to compare C$_2$ with C$_0$ monitoring [18]. However, the establishment of a C$_2$-monitoring program at Toronto was the result of an extensive review of pharmacokinetics and outcomes in a study performed by the Canadian Liver Transplant Group.

The Canadian Liver Transplant Study [3] was designed as a randomized, double-blind study to evaluate the effects of CsA formulation (Neoral vs. Sandimmune) on clinical outcomes. Patients with primary liver allografts ($n = 188$) were enrolled in this study. The secondary objective was a retrospective analysis comparing CsA pharmacokinetics with outcomes. Abbreviated AUC values for CsA were obtained for the first 6 h postdose in each of the study patients on days 5, 10, and 15 and week 16 following liver transplant. From this database, a maximum blood concentration of CsA was estimated (C$_{max}$). When subjects were categorized into quartiles based on the range of AUC$_{0-6}$ or C$_{max}$ values achieved, some significant correlations with acute rejection were observed. At week 2 posttransplant, the quartile group receiving Neoral with the highest C$_{max}$ value (>1200 ng/ml) exhibited the lowest mean incidence of acute rejection (31%) compared with the quartile group with the lowest C_{max} value (<600 ng/ml), which had an acute rejection incidence of 71%. Although this correlation between quartile and acute rejection was similar when AUC_{0-6} quartiles were identified, there was no such correlation when trough-level quartile groups were assessed.

The C_{max} value was confirmed as a surrogate marker of the abbreviated AUC, not only by direct correlation between parameters, but also by the similarity of clinical outcomes when both sets of quartiles were matched. Unfortunately, the C_{max} value is not the ideal practical tool for monitoring patients, as it is a value extrapolated from multiple blood samplings. However, the Neoral formulation provides an absorption pattern that is very consistent, and the 2-h post-dose sampling point (C_2) in this study cohort demonstrates an excellent correlation between C_{max} and C_2 in the de novo liver transplant patient. An important finding that resulted from this study was the identification of C_2 target levels for CsA in the de novo liver transplant patient [1]. Target C_2 levels were identified from months 0–6 (1.0 µg/ml) and for months 6–12 (0.8 µg/ml) posttransplant. These C_2 target recommendations were tested at Toronto General Hospital in 29 de novo liver transplant patients where CsA was initiated to achieve a target of 1.0 µg/ml within 3 days post-initiation of CsA dosing [19]. The incidence of acute rejection at 24 months posttransplant in this small pilot study was less than 15%. No increases in adverse events occurred compared with historical controls monitored by C_0, and the conclusions were that C_2 is a safe and effective monitoring tool in de novo liver transplant recipients.

The reliability of the C_2 sampling point as a tool for optimizing Neoral dosing in the de novo liver transplant patient has subsequently been tested and validated in a prospective, multicenter, open-label international study [18]. This study ($n = 307$) was designed to compare the utility of C_2 compared with C_0 for monitoring CsA therapy in liver transplantation. The target CsA range for the C_2 group ($n = 149$) between 0 and 3 months posttransplant was from 0.85 µg/ml to 1.40 µg/ml, and for the C_0 group ($n = 158$) it was from 250 ng/ml to 400 ng/ml for the same time-period.

At 3 months posttransplant, the C_2 group had a 25% reduction in the percentage of patients with acute rejection compared with the C_0 group (23.6% vs. 31%; $P = 0.06$). Of note, however, was the longer time the C_2-patient group took to achieve target levels, and this factor may have reduced the impact of C_2 on outcomes when compared with C_0. In those patients who achieved C_2 target levels by day 3 posttransplant, the acute rejection incidence was reduced to 12.5%. The incidence of moderate-to-severe acute rejection was significantly lower in the C_2-monitored group ($P = 0.01$) compared with the C_0 group (Fig. 7), but the tolerability and safety profiles were similar between treatment groups.

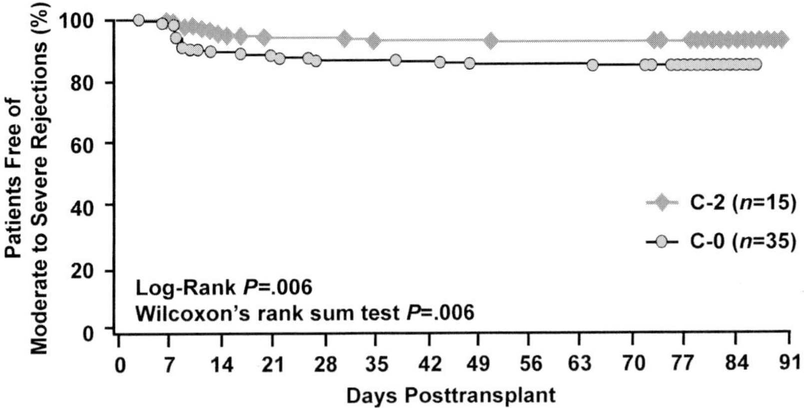

FIG. 7. Neoral C$_2$ monitoring results in a significant reduction in rejection severity (compared with C$_0$) in liver transplant recipients [18]

More recent studies were conducted at the University of Toronto to examine the effect of achieving C$_2$ targets (1.0 µg/ml) within 3–5 days on the incidence of rejection and renal function in de novo liver transplant recipients, and the effect of C$_2$-level monitoring on renal function in long-term patients treated with Neoral and who were being monitored by C$_0$ [20]. In 30 de novo patients, Neoral dosing was initiated at 15 mg/kg/day in divided doses, and adjustments to levels were made according to the formula:

$$\text{New dose} = \frac{\text{Old dose} \times \text{target level desired } (1.0\mu\text{g/l})}{\text{Level measured}}.$$

By day 3, 80% of patients achieved target, and by day 5, all patients achieved target using an aggressive dosing strategy as outlined above. No apparent renal toxicity was observed, with serum creatinine remaining within normal ranges (<110 µmol/l). An overall incidence of rejection of 7% (2/30 patients) was obse:ved, and in the two patients who suffered rejection, this was mild and was reversed by a single course of high-dose steroids.

One hundred long-term maintenance patients (mean 32 months posttransplant) on Neoral-based immunosuppression (monotherapy) and 64 patients on dual-therapy Neoral plus steroids (5 + 5 mg/day) were converted to C$_2$ monitoring. No correlation was observed between C$_0$ levels and C$_2$ levels. Furthermore, in several patients ($n = 28$) who had low levels of C$_0$ (50–100 ng/ml), high C$_2$ levels were observed (845 + 185 ng/ml). With a reduction in the dose, C$_2$ levels were lowered to a target of 600 ng/ml, which resulted in an improvement in renal function in all cases (from 164 + 45 µmol/l to 125 +

$20\,\mu mol/l$, $P < 0.01$). In other patients ($n = 55$), C_2 levels approximated recommended target levels ($600\,ng/ml$), although in a small number of patients ($n = 17$), C_2 levels were below target ($425 + 115\,ng/ml$) despite apparently adequate C_0 levels ($225 + 85\,ng/ml$). We elected to increase the dose of Neoral in these patients to achieve a target of $600\,ng/ml$ with no resultant adverse effect on renal function. In no cases did conversion to C_2 monitoring in these patients result in acute rejection, as evidenced by liver biochemistry, although no protocol biopsies were performed.

In summary, C_2 monitoring in the liver transplant recipient has been identified as a sensitive predictor of outcomes in a multicenter retrospective analysis. The Toronto General Hospital single-center prospective study demonstrated that C_2 monitoring is safe and effective. Finally, the international multicenter comparison between C_2 and C_0 validated C_2 as an effective monitoring tool in de novo liver transplant recipients.

Conclusions

The fundamental issue in CsA monitoring is that the traditional method of using predose trough, or C_0, CsA blood levels is not the most sensitive tool for the optimization of CsA immunosuppression in organ transplant recipients. Alternative monitoring strategies focused on the measurement of CsA exposure (or bioavailability) that utilized full AUC monitoring techniques. This approach, although documented as a sensitive predictor of clinical events in the transplant recipient, is cumbersome and expensive as a routine management tool.

Pharmacokinetic and pharmacodynamic data suggest that the absorption phase in the first $4\,h$ postdose is the zone of greatest individual variability, and may provide a sensitive and practical monitoring tool that has greater "differentiation" to determine the specific dosing needs of the individual patient. The abbreviated AUC_{0-4} monitoring method was identified as a sensitive predictor of selected clinical outcomes in renal transplant recipients, and prospective studies proved that the tool was effective in lowering acute rejection risk in de novo patients. The AUC_{0-4} method validated the use of CsA absorption measurements as being more effective than C_0 monitoring, but this approach still has the drawbacks of multiple sampling and subsequent analysis to derive a target level.

Two multicenter studies in de novo renal transplant patients demonstrated that the single sampling point at C_2 had the best correlation with AUC_{0-4} at all times tested posttransplant. Based on secondary analyses of these studies, a target C_2 level of $1.7\,\mu g/ml$ (mRIA analysis) was identified as optimal in the de novo renal transplant recipient. Subsequent target C_2 levels at later stages posttransplant and clinical validation through prospective studies are being

TABLE 1. Guidelines for Neoral target C$_2$ levels

Transplant recipient	Time posttransplant (months)	Target C$_2$ level (μg/ml)
Liver	0–6	1.0
	6–12	0.8
	12+	0.6
Renal	0–3	1.7
	3–6	1.2
	6–12	1.0
	12+	0.8

Target levels should be achieved within 3–5 days after starting Neoral therapy

planned, to provide further support for C$_2$ monitoring in renal transplant recipients.

C$_2$ monitoring in the liver transplant patient has been extensively researched because of two major multicenter studies that identified C$_2$ plus optimal target levels in the de novo patient, followed by a prospective multicenter study in more than 300 de novo patients that demonstrated the improvement in effectiveness of CsA immunosuppression with C$_2$ rather than C$_0$ monitoring. The patients monitored with C$_2$ therapy had a 25% reduction in acute rejection incidence and a significant reduction in rejection severity at 3 months posttransplant compared with patients monitored with C$_0$. This study not only provided clinical support for C$_2$ monitoring, but validated target levels for the de novo liver patient in the first 6 months posttransplant (Table 1).

Two aspects of C$_2$ monitoring have been identified that impact on the accuracy and utility of the monitoring method in general practice. First, there may be differences in sensitivity between analytical procedures for the determination of parent CsA concentrations. Investigations are in progress to determine the degree of change or conversion required for target C$_2$ levels using different assays. Second, sampling-time precision at 2 h postinitiation of the Neoral formulation dosing is the key to the accuracy of the C$_2$ method as a monitoring tool. Owing to the steep slope of the concentration–time curve during the absorption phase, variations in the sampling time will increase the variability in C$_2$ levels. Investigations are in progress to identify the span of time around the 2-h sampling point where accuracy is maintained.

In conclusion, CsA C$_2$ monitoring is a practical and sensitive method for monitoring CsA therapy. C$_2$ further maximizes immunosuppressive therapy compared with C$_0$ monitoring because it best reflects the absorption phase of CsA, which is the zone of greatest individual pharmacokinetic differentiation and period of maximal pharmacological effects. CsA C$_2$ target levels for renal and liver transplant recipients have been defined from prospective, multi-center clinical studies. Finally, C_2 monitoring has been validated as an effective monitoring tool in an international, multicenter, prospective study in liver transplant patients, and studies are ongoing to provide further support for C_2-monitoring methods in other transplant patient cohorts.

References

1. Belitsky P, Levy GA, Johnston A (2000) Neoral absorption profiling: an evolution in effectiveness. Transplant Proc 32(Suppl 3A):45S–52S
2. Mahalati K, Belitsky P, Sketris I, et al. (1999) Neoral monitoring by simplified sparse sampling area under the concentration-time curve: its relationship to acute rejection and cyclosporine nephrotoxicity early after kidney transplantation. Transplantation 68:55–62
3. Grant D, Kneteman N, Tchervenkov J, et al. (1999) Peak cyclosporine levels (C_{max}) correlate with freedom from liver graft rejection: results of a prospective, randomized comparison of Neoral and Sandimmune for liver transplantation (NOF-8). Transplantation 67:1133–1137
4. Lindholm A, Kahan BD (1993) Influence of cyclosporine pharmacokinetics, trough concentrations, and AUC monitoring on outcome after kidney transplantation. Clin Pharmacol Ther 54:205–218
5. Schroeder TJ, Hariharan S, First MR (1995) Variations in bioavailability of cyclosporine and relationship to clinical outcome in renal transplant subpopulations. Transplant Proc 27:837–839
6. Johnston A, David OJ, Cooney GF (2000) Pharmacokinetic validation of Neoral absorption profiling. Transplant Proc 32(Suppl 3A):53S–56S
7. Belitsky P, Dunn S, Johnston A, et al. (2000) Impact of absorption profiling on efficacy and safety of cyclosporin therapy in transplant recipients. Clin Pharmacokinet 39:117–125
8. Kahan BD (1989) Cyclosporine. N Engl J Med 321:1725–1738
9. Kahan BD, Welsh M, Schoenberg L, et al. (1996) Variable oral absorption of cyclosporine. A biopharmaceutical risk factor for chronic renal allograft rejection. Transplantation 62:599–606
10. Savoldi S, Maiorca R, Maderna M, et al. (1997) Low intra-patient variability of blood cyclosporine levels is correlated with excellent graft survival. Transplant Proc 29:288–289
11. Grevel J, Kahan BD (1991) Abbreviated kinetic profiles in area-under-the-curve monitoring of cyclosporine therapy. Clin Chem 37:1905–1908
12. Amante AJ, Kahan BD (1996) Abbreviated AUC strategy for monitoring cyclosporine microemulsion therapy in the immediate post-transplant period. Transplant Proc 28:2162–2163
13. Halloran PF, Helms LM, Kung L, et al. (1999) The temporal profile of calcineurin inhibition by cyclosporine in vivo. Transplantation 68:1356–1361
14. Sindhi R, LaVia MF, Paulling E (2000) Stimulated response of peripheral lymphocytes may distinguish cyclosporine effect in renal transplant recipients receiving a cyclosporine+rapamycin regimen. Transplantation 69:432–436 (abstract No. 12)
15. Keown P, Landsberg D, Halloran P, et al. (1996) A randomized, prospective multicenter pharmacoepidemiologic study of cyclosporine microemulsion in stable renal

graft recipients. Report of the Canadian Neoral Renal Transplantation Study Group. Transplantation 62:1744–1752
16. Mahalati K, Belitsky P, Kiberd B, et al. (2000) Absorption profiling—a novel method for monitoring Neoral in kidney transplantation that reduces rejection and nephrotoxicity. Transplantation 69(Suppl):S114 (abstract No. 12)
17. Barama A, Perner F, Beauregard-Zollinger L, et al. for the Neoral Phase IV Study Group (2000) Absorption profiling of cyclosporine therapy for de novo kidney transplantation: a prospective randomized study comparing sparse sampling to trough monitoring. Transplantation 69(Suppl):S162 (abstract No. 190)
18. Levy GA, Lake JR, Beauregard-Zollinger L, et al. for the Neoral Phase IV Study Group (2000) Improved clinical outcomes for liver transplant recipients using cyclosporine blood level monitoring based on two-hour post-dose levels. Transplantation 69(Suppl):S387 (abstract No. 1059)
19. Levy GA (1998) Neoral is superior to FK 506 in liver transplantation. Transplant Proc 30:1812–1815
20. Levy GA, O'Grady C, Lilly LB, et al. (2001) C-2 monitoring in liver transplantation with Neoral immunosuppression: Effect of achieving C-2 target early on efficacy and safety. Joint American Transplant Meeting; 2001: Chicago. Am J Transplant 1:310 (abstract No. 695)

The Interleukin 2 "Pathway" and the Route to Logical Immunosuppression

Björn Nashan

Summary. The interleukin (IL)-2/IL-2 receptor pathway plays a central role in the proliferation of T lymphocytes upon alloactivation. Since inhibition of the calcineurin/calmodulin complex is incomplete, IL-2 gene activation may occur, leading to IL-2 production and release. Animal models have demonstrated the efficacious synergism of calcineurin inhibitors such as cyclosporine and monoclonal antibodies targeting the α-chain of the IL-2 receptor to prevent acute rejection. The principle of immunoprophylaxis thus downregulates the immune cascades rather than eliminates lymphocytes, offering in theory the chance of logical immunosuppression without the burden of opportunistic infections or neoplasia. Large phase III clinical trials in renal and liver transplant recipients have demonstrated the proof of the principle. Immunoprophylaxis with IL-2 receptor inhibitors were side effect-free; i.e., no cytokine release syndrome was observed. The benefit of complementary immunosuppression achieved by the inhibition of the IL-2/IL-2 receptor pathway and the calcineurin/calmodulin complex resulted in increased efficacy. No increase in opportunistic infections, and particular in neoplasias, were observed. Thus complementary blockade of the IL-2 pathway is assumed to be a logical route to individually tailored immunosuppression.

Key words. Anti-IL-2 receptor monoclonal antibodies, Immunoprophylaxis, Complementary immunosuppression, Liver transplantation, Renal transplantation

---

Klinik für Viszeral- und Transplantationschirurgie, Medizinische Hochschule Hannover, Carl Neuberg Str. 1, 30625 Hannover, Germany

Introduction

The production of interleukin (IL)-2 plays a central role in the activation of T lymphocytes, and is an important initiation step in the whole process of the immune response to a transplanted organ [1, 2]. Although there are many signal pathways from the signalling caused by the antigen presentation on the surface of the T lymphocytes, calcineurin appears to feature on most of those pathways known to lead to IL-2 transcription and production in the cell nucleus [3]. This accounts for the excellent specificity and efficacy of calcineurin inhibitors such as cyclosporine. However, there appears to be a limit to the amount of calcineurin inhibition that can be realized in vivo, and this suggests that only about 50% inhibition can be obtained [4, 5]. This means that there is a further opportunity to block this "pathway" using specific treatments.

"Traditional" immunosuppression (antilymphocyte preparations, radiation, and splenectomy) aimed to reduce the immune response by removing the cells responsible for that response. This has fallen from favor, as these older methods tend to be nonselective and difficult to control. A new compound is now available which appears to offer physicians the ability to manipulate these cell populations, which may allow us to complement the control of the IL-2 pathway by modulation of the immune effector cells.

It has been realized for some time that the posttransplant period is a time of increased risk of rejection, and it has been associated with high blood levels of circulating IL-2. The IL-2 receptor (IL-2R) is pivotal for T cell activation, and is selectively expressed on activated T cells [6]. The IL-2R on the activated T lymphocyte is part of a "feed-forward" mechanism that, once stimulated, accelerates the immune response. An antibody that blocks this receptor seems a logical choice of treatment, and initial clinical trials were done with murine antibodies. The high-affinity IL-2R consists of three transmembrane protein chains termed α (CD25), β (CD122), and γ (CD132). The α chain is responsible for the rapid association of IL-2 with the β and γ chains to form the high-affinity receptor. Signal transduction is only possible by the high-affinity receptor or the combined β and γ chains. The α chain itself is not able to transduce signals due to its lack of a relevant cytoplasmic domain and it does not internalize [7–9], so blockade should not lead to the cytokine release syndrome seen with antibodies directed against other targets. Binding of a monoclonal antibody (mAb) to the α chain prevents formation of the high-affinity receptor and thus signal transduction. In the absence of immune stimulation, the α chain of the IL-2R is expressed in low amounts on CD4+, CD45RO+, CD4+, or CD45RA+ T cells [10]. Upon activation with antigen or mitogen, these cells enhance the expression of the α chain, which associates with the other components of the receptor to become the high-affinity receptor. In patients who were treated with a murine IL-2R mAb (BT563), the receptor was coated during the 12-day period of dosing, and IL-2R-positive cells belonged exclusively to the CD45R0+ subpopulation [10]. This suggests that specifically preactivated cells are coated, enabling rather selective and effective immunoprophylaxis in allografted patients.

Murine antibodies have a very short half-life in the body, so the murine antibody chosen for Simulect was chimerized with human immunoglobulin to extend its tolerability and longevity in the body. Pharmacokinetic data suggested that two doses of 20 mg would be sufficient to suppress CD25 for a period in excess of 30 days. This was felt to be sufficient to overcome the increased risk associated with the posttransplant period.

Simulect in Renal Transplantation

Two phase III, randomized, double-blind, placebo-controlled, multicenter trials were conducted in the USA and Europe/Canada to investigate basiliximab in combination with Neoral and steroids to prevent rejection in renal allograft recipients [11, 12]. Data from the studies were pooled, and the incidence of acute rejection, patient and graft survival, and safety and toleration were analyzed in the light of differences in patient demographics and management between the two trials. The two study protocols were similar. The patient demographics differed in that the US trial contained more Black patients and used living donors in approximately 30% of the cases. Patient management also differed owing to higher maintenance cyclosporin A (CsA) whole blood trough levels in the US study. A total of 728 patients undergoing primary renal transplantation were randomized to receive Simulect, 2×20 mg, or placebo. The first dose was given on the day of surgery and the second 4 days later. All patients received dual immunosuppressive therapy with Neoral and corticosteroids throughout the study period. The primary efficacy variable was a combined endpoint of death, graft loss, or acute rejection at 6 months posttransplant. Secondary efficacy variables included chronic or acute rejection, graft loss, and death, and safety and toleration from 6 to 12 months. Simulect treatment was associated with a 28.6% and 25.4% ($P < 0.001$) reduction in the combined incidence of death, graft loss, and rejection at 6 and 12 months, respectively. There were also significant reductions in the number of biopsy-confirmed rejection episodes. The reductions were also associated with a decreased use of steroids during the first month posttransplantation and the use of additional immunosuppressive agents. The results between the two studies were consistent despite differences in patient demographics and patient management. Simulect was effective in a variety of patient subgroups, irrespective of age, gender, ethnic origin, or donor type. Simulect treatment was well tolerated; the adverse event profile was comparable with that of the placebo, and there was no increase in the risk of infections. In conclusion, the addition of Simulect, 2b × 20 mg, to dual immunosuppressive therapy with Neoral and corticosteroids significantly reduced the incidence of acute rejection during the first year after renal transplantation. Patient tolerability of Simulect is comparable to that of placebo. The consistency of the pooled data with the USA and European/Canadian phase III trial results validates the results from the two studies and reinforces the conclusion that Simulect improves treatment outcomes in renal transplantation. Further subgroup analysis of the data indicates that Simulect has a beneficial effect in certain high-risk groups, in particular diabetics and patients under 50 years old. The evaluation of the USA data surprisingly indicated significantly better results in the living-relative donor group; this could imply that basiliximab is especially suitable for patients receiving grafts from relations.

An evaluation of 3-year results in one center (CHIB 201, Hannover, unpublished data) that included 41 (placebo $n = 20$, basiliximab $n = 21$) patients in the study showed 100% patient survival and a 95% and 90% graft survival with placebo and Simulect, respectively. Three grafts were lost (placebo $n = 1$, Simulect $n = 2$) due to technical complications. There was no difference in bacterial infections in the two groups, but patients on placebo had a significantly ($P = 0.02$) higher rate of cytomegalovirus (CMV) infections ($n = 5$) than those in the Simulect group ($n = 1$). Similarly, the distribution of acute rejections was 55% vs. 28.6% ($P < 0.05$). The placebo group had five steroid-resistant rejections, while there were none in the Simulect group. Thus, the cumulative amount of immunosuppression was higher in the placebo group, which is a possible explanation for the significantly higher rate of CMV infections. CsA trough levels started at 150 ng/ml and tapered to 110–120 ng/ml throughout the next 3 years. Creatinine values differed significantly after 3 years, i.e., 134 (±46) mmol/l in patients in the Simulect group and 175 (±53) mmol/l in patients in the placebo group ($P = 0.01$). After 3 years, no post-transplant lymphoproliferative disorders (PTLDs) or other malignancies were observed in any of the patients. According to this limited trial, basiliximab allow CsA to be used at roughly half the standard dose while still being effective, and resulting in a significantly improved function rate after 3 years in comparison to that of the placebo arm.

Further studies have demonstrated that Simulect remains efficacious when used in other regimens. In a 6-month, double-blind, placebo-controlled trial using triple therapy (with azathioprine), the Simulect group demonstrated a significant reduction in rejection rate to 20.8%. The study comprised 340 patients in 31 centers, and there was no difference in the frequency of adverse events between the two arms.

In a similar study, a 6-month, double-blind, placebo-controlled study of triple therapy with mycophenolate mofetil, the absolute rejection rate in the basiliximab arm was a very low 15.3%. This was another large study of 16 centers and 123 patients. Again there was no difference in the observed incidence of side effects between the two arms.

In conclusion, Simulect effectively reduces the incidence of acute rejection episodes in renal transplant recipients, with a low incidence of acute rejections in combination with Neoral and steroids, and a very low incidence of acute rejection in combination with Neoral and steroids, and azathioprine or mycophenolate mofetil. In all these studies there was no increase in the number of neoplasms in the Simulect arm compared with the placebo or active control arm. Thus, the incremental benefit of Simulect is maintained across maintenance regimens with a low incidence of death and graft loss.

Economic Implications of the Use of Simulect Versus Placebo in Renal Allograft Recipients

An economic evaluation was undertaken alongside the European/Canadian multicenter international phase III trial in renal transplant recipients [13]. The objectives of the study were to assess the within-trial resource usage and hence evaluate the cost implications of using Simulect and to explore how resource use relates to the clinical results, which were published separately. A total of 380 adult recipients of primary cadaveric kidney transplantation were recruited in seven countries throughout Europe and Canada. Patients were randomly allocated in this double-blind trial to receive a 20-mg infusion of basiliximab on the day of surgery and on day 4 to provide IL-2 receptor suppression for 4–6 weeks ($n = 193$), or to receive placebo ($n = 187$). All patients received dual-therapy maintenance immunosuppression with cyclosporine and steroids.

Secondary outcome measures included the occurrence of acute rejection and resource usage across several dimensions over the 12 months following transplantation. Local unit costs were obtained for each dimension, and a global trial analysis was facilitated by the use of health sector purchasing power parity (PPP) rates. The intention-to-treat analysis included 376 patients (Simulect $n = 190$, placebo $n = 186$). The study did not attempt to capture all of the costs of transplantation. Costs included were those that might vary with immunosuppression therapies. No statistically significant differences were found in any of the economically important categories of resource use or in the mean cost of treatment per patient, either across the whole trial or for any country. The mean cost of treatment (PPP $US), including the cost of Simulect, was $47 940 for Simulect patients (95% confidence interval [CI] $43 950–$51 920) and $46 280 for placebo patients (95% CI $42 280–$50 270). A country-level analysis indicated large differences between countries in resource usage and mean cost per patient. This suggests that there are very different treatment protocols and methods of working in operation within different countries. In conclusion, this international trial did not identify statistically significant results in terms of resource use and costs between Simulect and placebo, despite the clinical differences observed. The overall conclusion is that Simulect produces clinical benefit while the difference in the cost of treatment is not statistically significant. The average costs of treatment indicate that approximately 50% of the cost of the drug can be offset by reduced treatment costs. A similar study undertaken in the USA and reported elsewhere suggests that there is the potential for a complete offset of the drug costs. Treatment protocols within the countries included within this international study may prevent the full economic potential of Simulect being realized.

Pharmacokinetics and Pharmacodynamics of Simulect in Liver Transplantation

To improve the early postoperative course following liver transplantation the immunosuppressive effect as well as the disposition and pharmacokinetics of Simulect, were assessed in a prospective, open-label, phase I trial [14]. Focusing on pharmacokinetic and pharmacodynamic data, the primary objective was to investigate the impact of ascites fluid loss and blood loss on the bioavailability of Simulect. Twenty-four patients were enrolled in this study, of whom 23 received the full course of basiliximab. Basiliximab was given at a total of 40 mg either as 4×10 mg on days 0, 2, 4, and 6 ($n = 11$) or as 2×20 mg on days 0 and 4 ($n = 12$). Baseline immunosuppression consisted of cyclosporine (Neoral) and low-dose corticosteroids. Patients were followed for a total of 12 months. No clinically confirmed rejections occurred within the first 3 months after liver transplantation. Basiliximab was well tolerated, with no signs of a cytokine release syndrome or hypersensitivity. No CMV disease was observed. The 6 month survival rate was 92%; two patients died from septicemia (days 26 and 80) following complicated courses after bile duct necrosis and arterial thrombosis, respectively. The 12-month survival rate was 79%; one patient died from urosepsis (day 214), one from chronic ischemic bile duct damage and subsequent liver dysfunction (day 301), and one from hepatitis C reinfection (day 305). The central distribution volume was 5.6 ± 1.7l, indicating a slow body clearance of 75 ± 24 ml/h and an elimination half-life of 4.1 ± 2.1 days. Simulect was cleared at an average of 20% of total clearance via ascites fluid, where it was measurable. Total body clearance correlated positively with the volume of postoperative blood loss ($r = 0.5253$, $P = 0.01$), suggesting that bleeding may represent an additional route of drug removal. A threshold relation was observed between the serum concentration of Simulect and CD25 expression on T lymphocytes whereby complete saturation of the IL-2R α-chain was maintained as long as the serum concentration exceeded 0.1 µg/ml. CD25+ cells were coated with Simulect for 23 ± 7 days posttransplant (range 13–41 days). A two-dose regimen of Simulect proved to be safe and effective in liver allograft patients. These data provide preliminary evidence that therapy with the chimeric IL-2R mAb basiliximab reduces the incidence of acute rejection episodes, is well tolerated, and does not increase the occurrence of adverse events, in particular, viral or opportunistic infections.

Application of Simulect in Liver Transplant Recipients

Basing on these previous findings, a phase III, randomized, double-blind, placebo-controlled, multicenter trial was conducted in the USA, Canada, and Europe [15]. The ability of Simulect to improve the outcome in liver transplant recipients, as had been demonstrated for renal transplants, was assessed. A total of 381 adult recipients of a primary cadaveric liver transplantation were randomized to treatment, stratified by hepatitis C seropositivity. Patients received 40 mg of basiliximab ($n = 188$) or a placebo ($n = 193$) as two bolus injections of 20 mg on the day of surgery and 4 days later. Baseline immunosuppression consisted of cyclosporine and corticosteroids. Primary efficacy variables were biopsy-confirmed acute rejection and its composite endpoint, including death or graft loss, assessed at 6 and 12 months, and by hepatitis C virus (HCV) cohort. Following differential efficacy responses between HCV cohorts and clinical concern over HCV recurrence, an additional analysis incorporating HCV recurrence as a component of treatment failure, termed a "problem-free transplant," was introduced. Safety and tolerability were monitored over the 12 months of the study. Biopsy-confirmed acute rejection 6 months after transplantation was decreased in the basiliximab group. The reduction in rejection episodes was concentrated in the HCV-negative cohort, with a much smaller difference seen in the HCV-positive cohort. For HCV-positive patients, a "problem-free transplant" was demonstrated at 12 months in the basiliximab group as well as for all patients at 12 months. The incidence of infection and other adverse events was similar across the two treatment groups. As in the renal transplant population, no evidence of basiliximab-related side effects was noted. In summary, it was shown that immunoprophylaxis with 40 mg of basiliximab, in combination with cyclosporine and corticosteroids, reduces the incidence of acute rejection episodes, with no clinically relevant safety or tolerability concerns. The influence of HCV recurrence on the efficacy results can be accounted for in future trials by using the concept of a "problem-free transplant," incorporating recurrence as a component of treatment failure.

Conclusions

Simulect given in combination with maintenance immunosuppression (cyclosporine and steroids) obviously downregulates the main proliferation and differentiation pathways in CD25+ lymphocytes, a finding that is supported by experimental data [16]. These mechanisms are reversible, as was demonstrated by the increase in CD25 at the end of therapy indicating a release of the IL-2R signaling pathway. Although the IL-2R pathway has a central role in allograft rejection, IL-2R knockout mice reject islet cell allografts [17], and other cytokines such as IL-5 [18], IL-10 [19], and IL-15 [20] may play an important role in T cell-mediated rejection. An obvious difference between kidney and liver trials with IL-2R mAb is the difference in acute rejection rates. While in renal allografts an acute rejection incidence of 28%–35% [21–23] is observed, the incidence of acute rejections in liver-transplanted patients receiving a mAb ranges from less than 10% to 35% [24–27]. Apart from the difficult population of HCV-positive patients, in whom a clear-cut discrimination between HCV reinfection and acute rejection is not feasible, an explanation for this striking difference might be the different exposure to IL-15. IL-15 was initially cloned from a simian renal epithelial line [28], which implies that it might be constitutively expressed in human renal epithelial cells. Renal allograft patients might therefore have another potent cytokine that can circumvent the IL-2 pathway and is not inhibited in its action by cyclosporine [20].

Moreover data on IL-2 and γ-interferon in renal transplant patients support this hypothesis, since gene expression of both is necessary but not sufficient to lead to an acute rejection episode [29]. Macrophages/monocytes produce IL-15 as well, but so far there is no evidence that it is produced by liver cells. T cells could be exposed to different microenvironments depending on the allograft organ, and that might result in somewhat different activation patterns. Cyclosporine was given in low doses (CHIB 201, Hannover, unpublished data) [14], and the overall whole blood trough levels were around 150 ng/ml during the first weeks after transplantation. Similar cyclosporine levels have been reported in a previous trial [26] to be effective in combination with a murine IL-2R mAb (BT 563). In IL-2R mAb studies after liver transplantation in other groups [25, 27], cyclosporine trough levels were adjusted to 600–900 ng/ml [polyclonal assay, 27] and 250–300 ng/ml [monoclonal assay, 25]. Thus, first low cyclosporine trough levels in combination with IL-2 R mAb have a possible synergistic immunosuppressive effect in humans, and second, the advantage of this combination is the ability to avoid the nephrotoxicity of cyclosporine in the early posttransplant period.

The combination of both substances does not inevitably lead to excess immunosuppression with an increased risk of infections. In particular, trials using IL-2R mAb demonstrated the specific and restricted potential of this mAb as no increase in bacterial, viral, or mycotic infections was noted when murine, chimerized, or humanized mAbs (CHIB 201, Hannover, unpublished data) [11, 12, 21–27, 30, 31] were used. The incidence and course of infection following liver transplantation depend on the pretransplant clinical status as well as on the immunosuppression given. Thus, liver transplant patients are usually at a higher risk for infections. The low number of infections in these studies with no serious CMV disease supports this notion. The studies presented indicate that a combination of basiliximab with low-dose cyclosporine and steroids is associated with a low incidence of infections.

Because murine mAbs have short half-lives of between 24 and 48 h, and furthermore elicit a specific xenogeneic antibody response within the first week of application which leads to immunoelimination, attempts to chimerize or humanize mAbs have been carried out. Chimerized and humanized mAbs directed against IL-2R have already been used in phase I–III clinical trials in renal transplant patients [11, 12, 30, 31]. These trials demonstrated their superior biological function in terms of a long half-life and a xenogeneic antibody response in only a small number of patients. The lack of anti-idiotypic antibody responses in these studies extends the observations in renal transplantation to liver transplantation as well.

In conclusion, prophylactic immunosuppression with the IL-2R mAb Simulect given as a two-dose regimen, appears to be safe, well tolerated, and effective. Thus complementary blockade of the IL-2/IL-2R pathway is assumed to be a logical route to individually tailored immunosuppression.

References

1. Dendorfer U, Maslinksi W, Remillard B, et al. (1993) Interleukin-2 and the interleukin-2 receptor. Transplant Sci 3:83
2. Taniguchi T, Yasuhiro M (1993) The IL-2/IL-2 receptor system: a current overview. Cell 73:5
3. Ullman KS, Northrop JP, Verweij CL, et al. (1990) Transmission of signals from the T-lymphocyte antigen receptor to the genes responsible for cell proliferation and immune function: the missing link. Annu Rev Immunol 8:421

4. Batiuk TD, Pazderka F, Halloran PF (1995) Calcineurin activity is only partially inhibited in leukocytes of cyclosporine-treated patients. Transplantation 59:1400

5. Batiuk TD, Urmson J, Vincent D, et al. (1996) Quantitating immunosuppression. Estimating the 50% inhibitory concentration for in vivo cyclosporine in mice. Transplantation 6:1618

6. Morgan DA, Ruscetti FW, Gallo RC (19976) Selective in vitro growth of T-lymphocytes from normal human bone marrow. Sience 193:007

7. Kondo M, Takeshita T, Ishee N, et al. (1993) Sharing of the interleukin-2 (IL-2) receptor γ-chain between receptors for IL-2 and IL-4. Science 262:1874

8. Rusell SM, Keegan AD, Harada N, et al. (1993) Interleukin-2 receptor γ-chain: a functional component of the interleukin-4 receptor. Science 262:1880

9. Amlot PL, Tahami F, Chinn D, et al. (1996) Activation antigen expression on human T cells. I. Analysis by two-colour flow cytometry of umbilical cord blood, adult blood and lymphoid tissue. Clin Exp Immunol 105:176

10. Nashan B, Schwinzer R, Schlitt H, et al. (1995) Immunological effects of the anti-IL-2 receptor monoclonal antibody BT 563 in liver allografted patients. Transplant Immunol 3:203

11. Nashan B, Moore R, Amlot P, et al. (1997) Randomised trial of basiliximab versus placebo for control of acute cellular rejection in renal allograft recipients. Lancet 350:1193

12. Kahan BD, Rajagopalan PR, Hall M (1999) Reduction of the occurrence of acute cellular rejection among renal allograft recipients treated with basiliximab, a chimeric anti-interleukin-2-receptor monoclonal antibody. Transplantation 67:276

13. Chilcott J, Akehurst RL, Holmes M, et al. The economic implications of the use of basiliximab versus placebo for the prevention of acute cellular rejection in renal allograft recipients. Submitted for publication

14. Kovarik JM, Breidenbach Th, Gerbeau C, et al. (1998) Disposition and immunodynamics of basiliximab in liver allograft recipients. Clin Pharmacol Ther in press

15. Abstract at the AST 2000, Chicago, USA

16. Kupiec-Weglinski JW, Hahn HJ, Kirkman RL, et al. (1998) Cylcosporine potentiates the immunosuppressive effect of anti-interleukin 2 receptor monoclonal antibody therapy. Transplant Proc 20(suppl. 2):207

17. Steiger J, Nickerson PW, Steuer W, et al. (1995) IL-2 knockout recipient mice reject islet cell allografts. J Immunol 155:489

18. Martinez OM, Villnueva JC, Lake J, et al. (1993) Il-2 and Il-5 gene expression in response to alloantigen in liver allograft recipients and in vitro. Transplantation 55:1159

19. Xu GP, Sharma VK, Li B, et al. (1995) Intragraft expression of IL-10 messenger RNA: a noval correlate of renal allograft rejection. Kidney Int 48:1504

20. Pavlakis M, Strehlau J, Lipman M, et al. (1996) Intragraft IL-15 are increased in human renal rejection. Transplantation 62:543

21. Kirkman RL, Shapiro ME, Carpenter DB, et al. (1991) A randomized prospective trial of anti-Tac monoclonal antibody in human renal transplantation. Transplantation 51:107

22. Soulillou JP, Cantorovich D, LeMauff B, et al. (1990) Randomized controlled trial of monoclonal antibody against the interleukin-2 receptor (33B3.1) as compared with rabbit antithymocyte globulin for prophylaxis against rejection of renal allografts. N Engl J Med 322:1175

23. Amlot PL, Rawlings E, Fernando ON, et al. (1995) Prolonged action of a chimeric interleukin-2 receptor (CD25) monoclonal antibody used in cadaveric renal transplantation. Transplantation 60:748

24. Reding R, Feyaets A, Vraux H, et al. (1996) Prophylactic immunosuppression with anti-interleukin-2 receptor monoclonal antibody LO-Tact-1 versus OKT3 in liver allografting. A two-year follow-up study. Transplantation K61:1406
25. Neuhaus P, Bechstein WO, Blumhardt G (1993) Comparison of quadruple immunosuppression after liver transplantation with ATG or IL-2 receptor antibody. Transplantation 55:1320
26. Nashan B, Schlitt HJ, Schwinzer R, et al. (1996) Immunoprophylaxis with a monoclonal anti-IL-2 receptor antibody in liver transplant patients. Transplantation 61:546
27. Langrehr JM, Nüssler NC, Neumann U, et al. (1997) A prospective randomized trial comparing interleukin-2 receptor antibody versus antithymocyte globulin as part of a quadruple immunosuppressive induction therapy following orthotopic liver transplantation. Transplantation 63:1772
28. Giri J, Ahdieh M, Eisenman J, et al. (1994) Utilization of the β- and γ-chains of the IL-2 receptor by the novel cytokine IL-15. EMBO J 13:2822
29. McLean AG, Hughes D, Welsh KI, et al. (1997) Patterns of graft infiltration and cytokine gene expression during the first days of kidney transplantation. Transplantation 63:374
30. Vincenti F, Kirkman R, Light S, et al. (1998) Interleukin-2-receptor blockade with daclizumab to prevent acute rejection in renal transplantation. NEJM 338:161
31. Nashan B, Light S, Hardie IR, et al. (1999) Reduction of acute renal allograft rejection bz Daclizumab. Transplantation 67:110

FTY720: Mechanisms of Action and Immunosuppressive Activity in Organ Transplantation

SEIICHI SUZUKI

Summary. FTY720, a chemical substance derived by modifying an immunosuppressive metabolite from the ascomycete *Isaria sinclarii*, induces apoptosis specifically in lymphocytes and lymphocyte homing into lymphoid organs. After administration of the drug into liver-allografted rats at a dose of 0.5 mg/kg from day 1 to day 14 after grafting, the recipients survived significantly longer than those treated with no immunosuppressant. We showed that the drug induced proteolytic activation of caspases 2, 3, 6, 8, 9, and 10 in Jurkat cells, a human T lymphoma cell line, whereas caspases 1 and 5 were not activated. The caspase activation was initiated by cytochrome C released from mitochondria. Therefore, a broad caspase inhibitor prevented FTY720-induced apoptosis, but did not prevent cytochrome C release. In addition, the drug displays bcl-2-associated and Fas-independent apoptotic cell death. In canine kidney transplantation, the daily administration of FTY720 combined with cyclosporine resulted in remarkably prolonged graft survival in a synergistic manner. We also studied the combined effect of FTY720 with FK506 or gene therapy using a CTLA4Ig gene-containing adenovirus vector (adCTLA4Ig) in rat liver allografting. No adverse effects were observed in the drug-treated animals. Thus, FTY720 remains a promising drug for clinical application in the field of organ transplantation.

Key words. FTY720, Immunosuppressant, Caspase, Apoptosis, Cytochrome C

Department of Experimental Surgery and Bioengineering, National Children's Medical Research Center, 3-35-31 Taishido, Setagaya-ku, Tokyo 154-8509, Japan

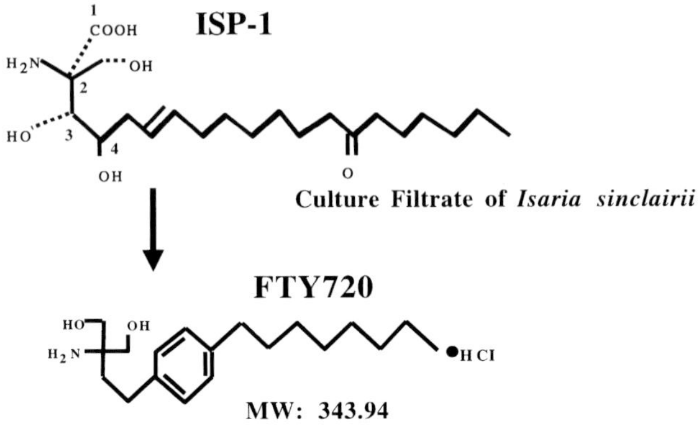

FIG. 1. Chemical structure of FTY720 and its original substance (ISP-1)

Introduction

Recently, immunosuppressive therapy has brought enormous advantages not only in the field of organ transplantation, but also in the treatment of allergic and autoimmune diseases. Current immunosuppressive drugs have some fundamental drawbacks: cyclosporine (CsA), tacrolimus (FK506), and other conventional drugs do not target only rejection-causing T cells, but also impair T cells protective against microorganisms. These immunosuppressants also cause metabolic derangement and organ toxicity even at their therapeutic doses. Therefore, a drug therapy that disables or eliminates only the T cells that respond specifically to donor antigens is desirable.

There is great interest in the recently developed immunosuppressant FTY720 (2-amino-[2-(4-octylphenyl)ethyl]-1,3-propanediol hydrochloride) [1]. FTY720 is a synthetic drug produced by the modification of ISP-1 purified from culture filtrates of *Isaria sinclairii*, an ascomycete (Fig. 1). The chemical structure and mechanism of action of FTY720 are completely different from those of conventional immunosuppressants [2].

Immunosuppressive Effect

Several groups have shown that FTY720 modifies lymphocyte homing receptors and/or adhesion molecules [3–5], although the drug triggers apoptosis specifically in lymphocytes and thus prevents allograft rejection without any severe side effects [6, 7]. As shown in Table 1, after the administration of FTY720 into liver-allografted rats at a dose of 0.5 mg/kg from day 1 to day 14 after transplantation, the recipients survived significantly longer than those treated with no immunosuppressant. In addition, pretransplant administra-

TABLE 1. Effects of FTY720 on liver allografts: prevention of graft rejection

Group	Survival days	Median
Control ($n = 10$)	$10 \times 2, 11 \times 3, 12 \times 3, 13, 15$	11.5
FTY720 ($n = 10$)	20, 22, 25, 26, 27, 28, 31, $37 \times 2, 47$	27.5

FTY720, 0.5 mg/kg p.o. on days 1–14

TABLE 2. Effects of FTY720 on liver allografts: effect on ongoing rejection

Groups	Survival days	Median
Control ($n = 12$)	$10 \times 2, 11 \times 4, 12 \times 3, 13,$ 14, 15	11.5
FTY720 ($n = 15$)	$13 \times 2, 15 \times 2, 21, 22, 24,$ 26, 28, 29, $30 \times 3, 31, 34$	26.0

FTY720, 5 mg/kg postoperatively on days 3 and 4

tion of FTY720 at 5 mg/kg one day before and on the day of grafting resulted in a remarkable prolongation of recipient survival [6, 8], and its administration at a same dosage on days 3 and 4 after grafting also prolonged survival (Table 2) [6, 9, 10].

To determine whether FTY720 induced apoptotic cell death in activated lymphocytes infiltrated into a grafted liver during acute rejection, we administered the drug at 5 mg/kg to recipients on day 3 and day 4 after grafting, when the graft rejection had been histologically confirmed. The treatment reversed ongoing rejection and significantly prolonged recipient survival time [11]. Light microscopic observation of the graft sections stained with the DNA nick-end labeling method showed that the apoptosis in the control allografts was mainly induced in hepatocytes, while that in the FTY720-treated allografts was in infiltrated lymphocytes. The rejection therapy with FTY720 did not alter the expressions of interleukin (IL)-2, interferon (IFN)-γ, and perforin mRNAs, but slightly decreased granzyme B expression. Thus, our results suggest that FTY720 does not alter the intrinsic lymphocyte function to produce the rejection-related cytokines, but strongly induces apoptotic cell death in the activated lymphocytes.

Using MRL-lpr/lpr mice (Fas antigen-mutant mice), we administered FTY720 for 14 days, beginning at 16 weeks of age, which was when the animals showed abnormally expanding lymphocytes [12]. MRL-lpr/lpr mice do not develop activation-induced cell death in lymphocytes owing to a congenital

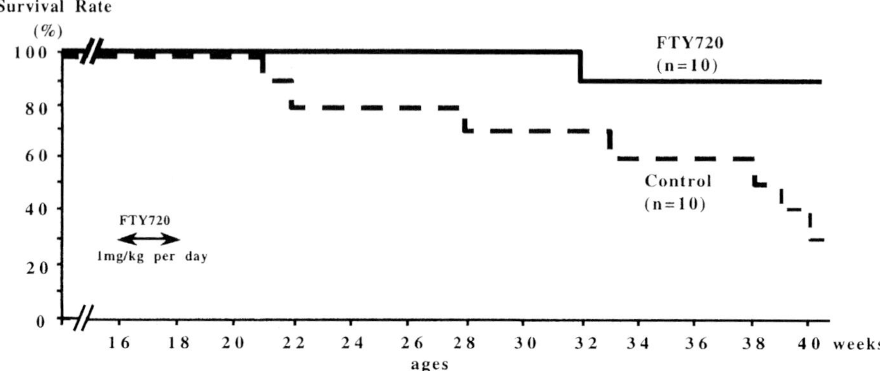

FIG. 2. Survival of MRL-lpr/lpr mice treated with FTY720, starting at 4 months of age, at a dose of 1 mg/kg for 14 days

defect of Fas antigen expression [13, 14]. We found a large number of TUNEL-staining cells in the thymus, spleen, and lymph nodes using the DNA nick-end labeling method. Furthermore, in vitro treatment with FTY720 resulted in dose-dependent cell death both in lpr-thymocytes and normal thymocytes. Although the mutant mice died from autoimmune disease, those treated with the drug survived significantly longer than the untreated mice (Fig. 2). Therefore, FTY720-induced apoptosis occurred in a Fas-independent manner.

Intracellular Events

Jurkat cells, a human T lymphoma cell line, transfected with bcl-2 gene were resistant to the drug. The intracellular ratio of Bcl-2 to Bax in human lymphocytes decreased immediately after the addition of FTY720 to the culture [15]. This suggests that FTY720 displays bcl-2-associated apoptotic cell death. Using HL-60 cells, a promyelocytoma cell line, FTY720 treatment induces apoptosis in these cells through phospholipase C activation and calcium mobilization from intracellular calcium pools [16]. Our recent study (manuscript in press) has indicated that treatment of Jurkat cells with FTY720 induced proteolytic activation of caspases 2, 3, 6, 8, 9, and 10, whereas caspases 1 and 5 were not activated. The treated cells also induced a loss of mitochondrial membrane potential, a release of cytochrome C into the cytosol, and an exposed phosphatidylserine at the outer surface of the cell membrane. Pretreatment with a broad caspase inhibitor prevented apoptosis and externalization of phosphatidylserine in the FTY720-treated cells, whereas this

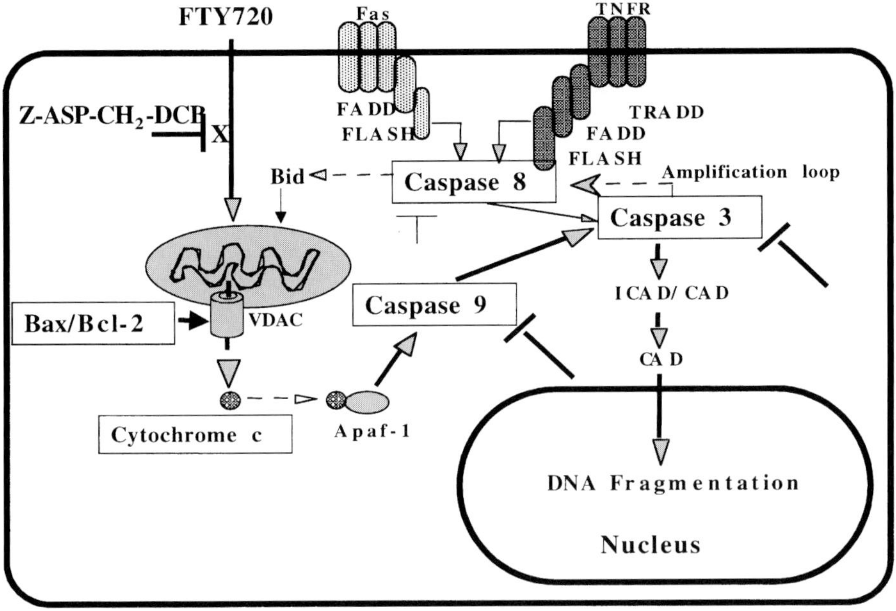

FIG. 3. Intracellular mechanisms of action of FTY720. *VDAC*, voltage-dependent anion channel (porin); *CAD*, caspase-activated DNAase; *ICAD*, inhibitor of CAD

inhibitor did not prevent the mitochondrial membrane potential or cytochrome C release. This suggests that caspases may play a role downstream from the mitochondrial pathway. These results indicate that the activation of caspases in FTY720-treated cells is initiated by cytochrome C released from mitochondria (Fig. 3).

Combination Therapy with Other Drugs

FTY720 in combination with CsA resulted in remarkably prolonged graft survival in canine kidney allografting [6, 17, 18]. Kahan and co-workers [19, 20] confirmed that FTY720 displays a synergistic interaction when combined with CsA and/or sirolimus in rat heart transplantation. We also found a combination effect between FTY720 and FK506 in rat liver allografting [21]. In addition, peritransplant administration of FTY720 in combination with posttransplant FK506 enhanced the survival of cardiac allografts in rats [8]. In these studies, FTY720 treatment did not produce animal morbidity or mortality.

TABLE 3. Effects of combination therapy with FTY720 and AdCTLA4Ig in rat heart transplantation

Group	n	Survival days	Median
Control	15	$5 \times 2, 6 \times 12, 7$	6
FTY720	12	$8 \times 5, 9 \times 4, 10, 13, 14$	9
AdCTLA4Ig	15	$20, 21, 22 \times 2, 24 \times 2, 27 \times 2, 28, 37, 38, 40, 42,$ 58, 62	27
FTY + AdCTLA4Ig	15	$21, 32, 33, 40, 42, 43, 54, 56, 65, 68, {>}100 \times 4$	56

AdCTLA4Ig, 1×10^9 plaque-forming units on day 0; FTY720, 5 mg/kg on day −1 and day 0

Combination Therapy with Gene Transfection

CTLA4Ig is a soluble recombinant fusion protein constructed with an extra-cellular domain of human CTLA4 and an Fc portion of human IgG1 [22]. It adheres strongly to B7 molecules on antigen-presenting cells and blocks CD28-mediated costimulatory signals in helper T cells [23, 24], which eventually inhibits immune responses to prolong graft survival in rodent models [25–29]. The administration of the CTLA4Ig-gene-containing adenovirus (adCTLA4Ig) via the tail vein into rats with cardiac allografts markedly prolonged graft survival times [30]. Furthermore, we performed adCTLA4Ig transfection combined with peritransplant administration of FTY720 in heart-grafted rats [31]. The median graft survival period in the adCTLA4Ig-alone group was 27 days, while that in the combination group was markedly prolonged to 56 days. It should be noted that five of 15 grafts survived indefinitely (Table 3). Thus, FTY720 and adCTLA4Ig have a potent mutual effect in prolonging allograft survival.

From these results, it can be seen that FTY720 remains a promising drug for combination with conventional immunosuppressants as well as gene therapy in the field of organ transplantation.

Conclusion

This chapter introduced the newly developed immunosuppressive drug FTY720. The mechanisms of its action have been reported to induce lymphocyte-specific apoptosis and lymphocyte homing into lymphoid organs. We have intensively investigated the intracellular mode of its action from the aspect of cell apoptosis. Interestingly, the drug produced no severe adverse reactions in rodents or dogs. In addition, it is of particular importance that FTY720 has a synergistic effect with CsA and FK506, which will be highly beneficial if clinical trials are considered in the future. A phase I clinical study has already been completed with satisfactory results, and a phase

II study is now ongoing in European countries and the United States. The final goal of allogeneic organ grafting will be the induction of transplantation tolerance. By using FTY720 in combination with other conventional immunosuppressants or gene therapy, we should achieve that goal in the near future. This is a novel strategy for clinical transplantation in the 21st century.

References

1. Fujita T, Yoneta M, Hirose, R, et al. (1995) Simple compounds, 2-alkyl-2-amino-1,3-propanediols, have potent immunosuppressive activity. Bioorg Med Chem Lett 5: 847–853
2. Baumann G (1992) Molecular mechanism of immunosuppressive agents. Transplant Proc 24:4–7
3. Chiba K, Yanagawa Y, Masubuchi Y, et al. (1998) FTY720, a novel immunosuppressant, induces sequestration of circulating mature lymphocytes by acceleration of lymphocyte homing in rats. I. FTY720 selectively decreases the number of circulating mature lymphocytes by acceleration of lymphocyte homing. J Immunol 160:5037–5044
4. Yanagawa Y, Sugahara K, Kataoka H, et al. (1998) FTY720, a novel immunosuppressant, induces sequestration of circulating mature lymphocytes by acceleration of lymphocyte homing in rats. II. FTY720 prolongs skin allograft survival by decreasing T cell infiltration into grafts but not cytokine production in vivo. J Immunol 160:5493–5499
5. Li XK, Enosawa S, Kakefuda T, et al. (1997) FTY720, a novel immunosuppressive agent, enhances upregulation of the cell adhesion molecular ICAM-1 in TNF-alpha-treated human umbilical vein endothelial cells. Transplant Proc 29:1265–1266
6. Suzuki S, Enosawa S, Kakefuda T, et al. (1996) A novel immunosuppressant, FTY720, with a unique mechanism of action, induces long-term graft acceptance in rat and dog allotransplantation. Transplantation 61:200–205
7. Suzuki S, Enosawa S, Kakefuda T, et al. (1996) Long-term graft acceptance in allografted rats and dogs by treatment with a novel immunosuppressant, FTY720. Transplant Proc 28:1375–1376
8. Xu M, Antoniou EA, Afford SC, et al. (1997) Effect of peritransplant FTY720 alone or in combination with posttransplant FK506 in a rat model of cardiac allotransplantation. Transplant Proc 29:2964–2966
9. Suzuki S, Enosawa S, Kakefuda T, et al. (1996) Immunosuppressive effect of new drug, FTY720, on lymphocyte response in vitro and cardiac allograft survival in rats. Transplant Immunol 4:252–255
10. Xu M, Pirenne J, Antoniou S, et al. (1998) FTY720 compares with FK506 as rescue therapy in rat heterotopic cardiac transplantation. Transplant Proc 30:2221–2222
11. Li X-K, Tamura A, Fujino M, et al. (2001) Induction of lymphocyte apoptosis in rat liver allograft with ongoing rejection by FTY720. Clin Exp Immunol 123:331–339
12. Suzuki S, Li X-K, Shinomiya T, et al. (1997) The induction of lymphocyte apoptosis in MLR-lpr/lpr mice treated with FTY720. Clin Exp Immunol 107:103–111
13. Cohen PL, Eisenberg RA (1991) Lpr and gld: single-gene models of systemic autoimmunity and lymphoproliferative disease. Annu Rev Immunol 9:243–269
14. Hang L, Theofilopoulos AN, Dixon F (1982) A spontaneous rheumatoid arthritis-like disease in MRL/l mice. J Exp Med 155:1690–1701
15. Suzuki S, Li X-K, Enosawa S, Shinomiya T (1996) A new immunosuppressant, FTY720, induces bcl-2-associated apoptotic cell death in human lymphocytes. Immunology 89:518–523

16. Shinomiya T, Li X-K, Amemiya H, et al. (1997) An immunosuppressive agent FTY720 increases intracellular concentration of calcium ion and induces apoptosis in HL60. Immunology 91:594–600
17. Suzuki S, Enosawa S, Kakefuda T, et al. (1996) Long-term graft acceptance in allografted rats and dogs by treatment with novel immunosuppressant, FTY720. Transplant Proc 28:1375–1376
18. Suzuki S, Kakefuda T, Amemiya H, et al. (1998) An immunosuppressive regimen using FTY720 combined with cyclosporin in canine kidney transplantation. Transplant Int 11:95–101
19. Stepkowski SM, Wang M-E, Qu X, et al. (1998) Synergistic interaction of FTY720 with cyclosporine or sirolimus to prolong heart allograft survival. Transplant Proc 30: 2214–2216
20. Wang M-E, Tejpal N, Qu X, et al. (1998) Immunosuppressive effects of FTY720 alone or in combination with cyclosporine and/or sirolimus. Transplantation 65:899–905
21. Tamura A, Li X-K, Funeshima N, et al. (2000) Immunosuppressive therapy using FTY720 combined with tacrolimus in rat liver transplantation. Surgery 127:47–54
22. Linsley PS, Brady W, Urnes M, et al. (1991) CTLA-4 is a second receptor for the B cell activation antigen B7. J Exp Med 174:561–569
23. Wu Y, Guo Y, Liu Y (1993) A major costimulatory molecule on antigen-presenting cells, CTLA4 ligand A, is distinct from B7. J Exp Med 178:1789–1793
24. Lenschow DJ, Zeng Y, Thistlethwaite JR, et al. (1992) Long-term survival of xenogeneic pancreatic islet grafts induced by CTLA4Ig. Science 257:789–792
25. Turka LA, Linsley PS, Lin H, et al. (1992) T-cell activation by the CD28 ligand B7 is required for cardiac allograft rejection in vivo. Proc Natl Acad Sci USA 89:11102–11105
26. Sayegh MH, Zheng X-G, Magee C, et al. (1997) Donor antigen is necessary for the prevention of chronic rejection in CTLA4Ig-treated murine cardiac allograft recipients. Transplantation 64:1646–1650
27. Pearson TC, Alexander DZ, Corbascio M, et al. (1997) Analysis of the B7 costimulatory pathway in allograft rejection. Transplantation 63:1463–1469
28. Glysing-Jensen T, Raisanen-Sokolowski A, Sayegh MH, et al. (1997) Chronic blockade of CD28-B7-mediated T-cell costimulation by CTLA4Ig reduces intimal thickening in MHC class 1 and 2 incompatible mouse heart allografts. Transplantation 64:1641–1645
29. Lin H, Bolling SF, Linsley PS, et al. (1993) Long-term acceptance of major histocompatibility complex mismatched cardiac allografts induced by CTLA4Ig plus donor-specific transfusion. J Exp Med 178:1801–1806
30. Kita Y, Li X-K, Ohba M, et al. (1999) Prolonged cardiac allograft survival in rats systemically injected adenoviral vectors containing CTLA4Ig-gene. Transplantation 68:758–766
31. Ohba M, Li X-K, Kita Y, et al. (2001) The combined therapy of CTLA4Ig-gene transfection with FTY720: FTY720 may enhance the effect of gene therapy. World J Surg 24:115–124

Novel Strategies for Living Donor Liver Transplantation Across the ABO Blood Group Barrier: Effect of Intraportal Infusion Therapy

Minoru Tanabe, Motohide Shimazu, Go Wakabayashi, Ken Hoshino, Yasuhide Morikawa, and Masaki Kitajima

ABO-incompatible liver transplantation is associated with an extremely complicated postoperative course, especially when the recipients are adults and older children. The recipient's preexisting antibody for donor-blood-group antigen induces serious rejection with a high incidence biliary and vascular complications. We had two cases of successful adult living donor liver transplantation across the ABO blood group barrier using intraportal infusion therapy, a novel antirejection regimen. Patient 1 was a 52-year-old woman with primary biliary cirrhosis (blood group O). She underwent living donor liver transplantation on November 16, 1998, using the left lobe graft from her son (blood group A). Patient 2 was a 45-year-old man referred with subacute hepatic failure of unknown etiology (blood group A). Living donor liver transplantation was performed on June 4, 2000, using a right lobe graft from his younger brother (blood group AB). Preoperatively, antidonor blood group antibody was removed by multiple plasmaphereses, and cyclophosphamide was administered for immunosuppression. Splenectomy was performed during transplantation; and tacrolimus, steroids, and cyclophosphamide were given postoperatively for basic systemic immunosuppression. In addition to these conventional therapies, methylprednisolone, prostaglandin E_1, and gabexate mesylate were infused postoperatively from the graft portal vein catheter that had been inserted during the operation. Initial graft function in the first case was fairly good, but she developed an intraabdominal hematoma 12 days after transplantation that required hemostasis during relaparotomy. Obstructive jaundice and cholangitis appeared during the third week after transplantation but were successfully managed by temporary percataneous transhepatic cholangrographic drainage and administration of antibiotics. Cytomegalovirus (CMV) antigenemia was detected but without significant

Department of Surgery, School of Medicine, Keio University, 35 Shinanomachi, Shinjuku-ku, Tokyo 160-8582, Japan

symptoms during the third week after transplantation; but the test reverted to negative with ganciclovir treatment. She was discharged 73 days after transplantation. The postoperative course of the second case was not problematic during the first 2 weeks after transplantation, and initial graft function was satisfactory. Biliary anastomotic leakage became evident (duct-to-duct anastomosis) the third week after transplantation and was resolved conservatively. He complained of dull pain on the upper abdomen during the ninth week after transplantation, which was diagnosed as CMV colitis by colonoscopy. The colitis was treated successfully with ganciclovir therapy. He was discharged 131 days after transplantation. Neither patient showed any vascular complications or rejection throughout the postoperative course. Biliary complications were temporary and resolved completely. These patients have now survived 27 and 8 months after transplantation, respectively. Their graft functions and general conditions are quite good, and they are enjoying normal, healthy lives.

Key Word Index